House on Fire

CALIFORNIA/MILBANK BOOKS ON HEALTH AND THE PUBLIC

1. *The Corporate Practice of Medicine: Competition and Innovation in Health Care,* by James C. Robinson
2. *Experiencing Politics: A Legislator's Stories of Government and Health Care,* by John E. McDonough
3. *Public Health Law: Power, Duty, Restraint,* by Lawrence O. Gostin (revised and expanded second edition, 2008)
4. *Public Health Law and Ethics: A Reader,* edited by Lawrence O. Gostin (revised and updated second edition, 2010)
5. *Big Doctoring in America: Profiles in Primary Care,* by Fitzhugh Mullan, M.D.
6. *Deceit and Denial: The Deadly Politics of Industrial Pollution,* by Gerald Markowitz and David Rosner
7. *Death Is That Man Taking Names: Intersections of American Medicine, Law, and Culture,* by Robert A. Burt
8. *When Walking Fails: Mobility Problems of Adults with Chronic Conditions,* by Lisa I. Iezzoni
9. *What Price Better Health? Hazards of the Research Imperative,* by Daniel Callahan
10. *Sick to Death and Not Going to Take It Anymore! Reforming Health Care for the Last Years of Life,* by Joanne Lynn
11. *The Employee Retirement Income Security Act of 1974: A Political History,* by James A. Wooten
12. *Evidence-Based Medicine and the Search for a Science of Clinical Care,* by Jeanne Daly
13. *Disease and Democracy: The Industrialized World Faces AIDS,* by Peter Baldwin
14. *Medicare Matters: What Geriatric Medicine Can Teach American Health Care,* by Christine K. Cassel
15. *Are We Ready? Public Health since 9/11,* by David Rosner and Gerald Markowitz
16. *State of Immunity: The Politics of Vaccination in Twentieth-Century America,* by James Colgrove
17. *Low Income, Social Growth, and Good Health: A History of Twelve Countries,* by James C. Riley
18. *Searching Eyes: Privacy, the State, and Disease Surveillance in America,* by Amy L. Fairchild, Ronald Bayer, and James Colgrove
19. *The Health Care Revolution: From Medical Monopoly to Market Competition,* by Carl F. Ameringer
20. *Real Collaboration: What It Takes for Global Health to Succeed,* by Mark L. Rosenberg, Elisabeth S. Hayes, Margaret H. McIntyre, and Nancy Neill
21. *House on Fire: The Fight to Eradicate Smallpox,* by William H. Foege
22. *Inside National Health Reform,* by John E. McDonough

House on Fire

THE FIGHT
TO ERADICATE SMALLPOX

WILLIAM H. FOEGE

University of California Press
BERKELEY   LOS ANGELES   LONDON

Milbank Memorial Fund
NEW YORK

University of California Press
Berkeley and Los Angeles, California

University of California Press, Ltd.
London, England

© 2011 by The Regents of the University of California

First paperback printing 2012

Library of Congress Cataloging-in-Publication Data

Foege, William H., 1936–.
    House on fire : the fight to eradicate smallpox / William H. Foege.
        p.   cm — (California/Milbank books on health and the public ; 21)
    Includes bibliographical references and index.
    ISBN 978-0-520-27447-1 (pbk. : alk. paper)
    1. Smallpox.   I. Milbank Memorial Fund.   II. Title.   III. Series: California/
Milbank books on health and the public ; 21.
    [DNLM: 1. Smallpox—epidemiology—Africa—Personal Narratives.
2. Smallpox—epidemiology—India—Personal Narratives.   3. History, 20th
Century—Africa—Personal Narratives.   4. History, 20th Century—India—
Personal Narratives.   5. International Cooperation—Africa—Personal
Narratives.   6. International Cooperation—India—Personal Narratives.
7. Smallpox—history—Africa—Personal Narratives.   8. Smallpox—history—
India—Personal Narratives.   WC 585]
    RA644.S6F64   2011
    614.5'21—dc22   2010041703

Manufactured in the United States of America

20
10 9 8 7 6 5 4 3

To my wife, Paula, for making this work even possible;
to Patty Stonesifer, for the support that made it possible to
write the account; and to the legions, from WHO/Geneva
to households around the world, who made smallpox
eradication a reality

If a house is on fire, no one wastes time putting water on nearby houses just in case the fire spreads. They rush to pour water where it will do the most good— on the burning house. The same strategy turned out to be effective in eradicating smallpox.

Contents

List of Illustrations   xi

Foreword by Carmen Hooker Odom and Samuel L. Milbank   xiii

Foreword by David J. Sencer   xv

Preface   xix

PART ONE   AFRICA: IDENTIFYING THE KEY STRATEGY

1. A Loathsome Disease   3

2. A Succession of Mentors   12

3. Practicing Public Health in Nigeria   28

4. Fire Line around a Virus   43

5. Extinguishing Smallpox in a Time of War   60

PART TWO   INDIA: MEETING THE CHALLENGE
            OF ERADICATION

6. Under the Rule of Variola   83

7. Unwarranted Optimism   105

8. A Gorgeous Coalition   123

9. Rising Numbers, Refining Strategy   145

10. Water on a Burning House   163

11. Smallpox Zero   173

    Conclusion   188

    Postscript   193

    Appendix: A Plan in the Event of Smallpox Bioterrorism   195

    Notes   199

    Glossary   209

    Index   213

Illustrations

FIGURES

1. Statue of Edward Jenner vaccinating a child   9
2. David Foege and village children, Nigeria, 1965   35
3. Rotary lancet, a vaccination device used in India until the
   early 1970s   50
4. Ped-O-Jet, the delivery instrument for millions of vaccinations
   in Africa in the 1960s   51
5. First smallpox patient seen in Ogoja, Nigeria, outbreak, 1966   55
6. Patient outside infectious disease hut near Abakaliki, Nigeria, 1967   58
7. The first cadre of smallpox warriors, Ghana, 1967   70
8. A village smallpox goddess   90
9. The bifurcated needle   101
10. Search team member in India seeking information on
    smallpox using a recognition card   109

11. Smallpox reports from weeks 34 to 47 in Uttar Pradesh and
    Bihar, India, 1973   116

12. Average number of new and contained outbreaks per week,
    Bihar, India, January to April 1974   148

13. Average number of new and contained outbreaks per week,
    Bihar, India, January to May 1974   164

14. Graph distributed to field-workers showing the turning point,
    when outbreaks began to decrease in India, 1974   174

15. Total outbreaks per week in India, January 1974 to May 1975   184

16. Instructions given to field-workers for vaccinating with
    the bifurcated needle   197

TABLE

1. Smallpox deaths in well-vaccinated British India, 1868–1907   96

MAPS

1. Nigeria, 1966–67   31

2. Northern India   106

3. New smallpox outbreaks in Bihar, India:
   1974 and 1975 compared   178

Foreword

CARMEN HOOKER ODOM, *President, Milbank Memorial Fund*
SAMUEL L. MILBANK, *Chairman, Milbank Memorial Fund*

The Milbank Memorial Fund is an endowed operating foundation that works to improve health by helping decision makers in the public and private sectors acquire and use the best available evidence to inform policy for health care and population health. The Fund has engaged in nonpartisan analysis, study, research, and communication since its inception in 1905.

House on Fire: The Fight to Eradicate Smallpox, by William H. Foege, is the twenty-first book in the series California/Milbank Books on Health and the Public. The publishing partnership between the Fund and the University of California Press encourages the synthesis and communication of findings from research and experience that could contribute to more effective health policy.

With an insider's knowledge of the worldwide smallpox eradication program in the 1960s and 1970s, Foege, a physician, relates the strategies used to eradicate smallpox in Africa and India and the challenges encountered along the way. He reveals the reasons behind the success of this program: a shared global objective; conception, implementation, and management of a clear plan tailored to a specific disease in terms of its context, range, and vulnerabilities; evaluation of the tools and techniques used and their subsequent modification; a willingness at all levels, from the local citizenry and government to country officials and global institutions, to communicate and work together to achieve the end goal; tenacity; and optimism.

As Foege notes, the smallpox eradication program shows that "humanity does not have to live in a world of plagues, disastrous governments, conflict, and uncontrolled health risks. The coordinated action of a group of dedicated people can plan for and bring about a better future. The fact of smallpox eradication remains a constant reminder that we should settle for nothing less."

This book should be useful to policymakers, foundations, and nongovernmental service organizations as well as to professionals in global health as they work together to confront the shared global risk of emerging and reemerging infectious diseases.

Foreword

DAVID J. SENCER

The eradication of smallpox from the entire world has been justly described as one of the most remarkable achievements in the history of medicine and public health. In India—a country one-third the size of the United States but with three times the population, with 638,365 villages and thirty-five cities with a million-plus population—the campaign to eradicate smallpox involved the most acute and challenging difficulties encountered anywhere in the entire smallpox eradication effort. The story of India's successful eradication program can be told fully only by those who were on the team that brought about this achievement, and this book is written by one of the team's two pivotal participants. It is so much richer because this participant happens to have one of the most impressive memories in the world, and he has used his own extensive notes and references from others involved in the campaign.

The other pivotal participant, Dr. M. I. D. Sharma, was the director of the smallpox eradication program for the Government of India during the years when this final effort was mounted and brought to a successful conclusion in 1975. He also served concurrently as the director of India's National Institute of Communicable Diseases. His unflagging commitment to eradication, the excellence of his leadership, and his skillful use of the human, fiscal, and material resources—committed from all over the world—in the Indian eradication effort constituted a central and indispensable element in the success of this program.

Dr. William Foege, as a Centers for Disease Control and Prevention (CDC) epidemiologist assigned to the Southeast Asia Regional Office of the World Health Organization (WHO), worked on the eradication effort throughout the Indian subcontinent. The methodology of surveillance and containment, an alternative to mass vaccination refined in the 1960s in Africa, enabled the Indian and multinational team to successfully eradicate smallpox in India. Dr. Foege's tenacious advocacy of the containment approach, together with his meticulous monitoring of the continually changing status of the Indian eradication effort and his adjustment of strategy and resources in response to altered circumstances, was an essential ingredient of this success.

Much has been said about the humanitarian benefits derived from the eradication of smallpox, and the importance of these benefits to all the nations of the world cannot be disputed. But another benefit of almost equal weight in the minds of many public health professionals was the demonstration that the Indian government and its people could apply principles of sound management and deliver a program that stretched from the remotest village to the most populous urban centers of their country. Supervision, delegation, evaluation, performance appraisal, and accountability—all commonplace terms in the business schools of the world—acquired operational reality in this vast undertaking. The concepts and practices of sound management became a reality in the work of more than 250,000 workers throughout the nation.

The health and well-being of people throughout the world have been enhanced by the dedication of these Indian smallpox eradication workers, by the responsiveness of the hundreds of millions of Indian people who accepted vaccination and actively collaborated in the reporting of disease and suspected cases, and by the hundreds of health workers from other nations who, with their Indian counterparts, devoted the best of their skills and capacities to this effort. All of us, and those who will follow us, are indebted to these workers and to their leaders, particularly to the late Dr. Sharma and those who collaborated so closely and effectively with him in this last major battle of the war against smallpox.

The author of this volume was in a delicate position in India. Dr. Foege was recognized by the Indian leadership as a representative of WHO and the CDC, but his precise role and scope of responsibilities in the eradication effort were not crisply defined. He had to persuade the authorities to make necessary changes and to recognize that eradication was achievable only if the CDC continued to provide the resources needed. Dr. Foege demonstrated to all levels of the Indian bureaucracy qualities of leadership that often go unrecognized. For one thing, he was willing to do whatever it took for the effort to continue. It was not unusual for him to place himself in physical jeopardy for the sake of the program. For example, he would carry millions of rupees in his briefcase to make sure that payrolls were met. Some people believe that leadership means being out in front, being visible; Dr. Foege demonstrated that great leaders can lead from behind the scenes, giving others the credit and recognition.

The publisher and a number of colleagues urged Dr. Foege to place himself more visibly in the narrative. But the publisher does not know Dr. Foege. As director of the CDC, I was one of his supervisors while he was working on smallpox eradication in India, and I have known him for more than forty years. He tells stories not about what he has done, but about what others have done. Dr. Foege called me from India about six months before the last case of smallpox was contained. I urged him to remain there and asked whether he realized that in a few months, the last case of smallpox in India would be eradicated and that there would be a huge celebration for one of the most extraordinary events in the history of global health. He responded, "I realize that this is going to happen, but if I remain in India, too much attention would be directed toward the external support that India received, and it is very important that recognition be given to the accomplishments of the hundreds of thousands of Indians who really did the work." He said to me, "This is why I am coming home." And against my suggestion, he packed up, and he and his family came home.

This principle of "ego suppression" continued to guide Dr. Foege as he returned to the United States and pursued his lifelong career goal of working as the director of the CDC, as the founder of the Task Force for Child Survival, as the executive director of the Carter Center, and as a senior advisor to the Bill and Melinda Gates Foundation, all in the pursuit of global health equity. The world's debt to William Foege is enormous.

Preface

We lose our histories far too fast. In the dozens of public health efforts in which I have been involved throughout my career, the histories have rarely been written soon enough. Within years, sometimes within months, people's accounts begin to differ. Often the participants simply do not keep journals or record their notes. In an effort to capture the history of the smallpox eradication effort forty years after the fact, the participants at the 2006 reunion of the first smallpox workers sent by the Centers for Disease Control and Prevention (CDC) in Atlanta to West and Central Africa in the mid-1960s were invited to record oral histories. Many commented that they had forgotten details, and their accounts were incomplete. Based on this experience, the CDC decided to collect oral histories from the people involved in the 2010 H1N1 influenza phenomenon right away, in 2010. This is a wise practice, for much that might benefit future generations can be learned from eyewitness accounts of important events.

Thousands of people participated in the global smallpox eradication effort in the 1960s and 1970s, and each one has a story to tell. Their stories might vary, yet the people involved shared common attributes. They were optimists; they actually thought they could change the future—and they did. They were risk takers; there was no shortage of people telling them that the effort was futile and they were hurting their career chances—this proved untrue. They were problem solvers; they had little idea of what they were facing, and they took on the problems in order and in stride. They also knew how to mix hard work and fun. Working under sometimes grueling conditions in hot and humid village regions worldwide, with few amenities, these field-workers gathered periodically for meetings where humor and the shared sense of being part of something important carried the day.

This book tells the story of one of those workers, and, like the accounts of any single team member, it is subject to memory defects, biases, and faulty interpretations. One advantage is that I was involved in the eradication effort from the beginning. I did keep rudimentary notes, but errors in my account are probable and I am responsible for them.

My gratitude goes first to the countless workers around the world who achieved smallpox eradication. I am especially grateful for my colleagues in India, including Drs. P. Diesh, M. I. D. Sharma, Mahendra Dutta, and C. K. Rao. There is no way to adequately thank the World Health Organization (WHO) and CDC people I worked with: in New Delhi, especially Drs. Nicole Grasset, Zdeno Jezek, Larry Brilliant, Don Francis, Don Hopkins, Prem Gambhiri, and Harcharn Singh; in Geneva, the WHO staff, led by D. A. Henderson; and in Atlanta and around the world, the CDC workers, especially Dave Sencer, Bill Watson, Stu Kingma, Don Millar, Bill Griggs, Stan Foster, Joan Davenport, Jeff Koplan, Don Eddins, Frances Porcher, Ann Mather, Maudine Ford, and Carol Walters—and at least one hundred others.

Countless colleagues in Nigeria helped make the early days productive. These include Wolfgang Bulle, David Thompson, Paul Lichfield, and the missionaries who helped during the first smallpox outbreak in Ogoja, among them Annie Voigt, Hector Ottemüller, Harold Meissner, and Wally Rasch. The support staff in Lagos included George Lythcott, Rafe Henderson, Jim Hicks, and Stan Foster.

Institutions help provide the structure, the resources, and the ability to develop objectives, coalitions, and programs. I am especially thankful for the support and assistance of the Centers for Disease Control and Prevention, the Carter Center, Emory University, and the Bill and Melinda Gates Foundation. It is an honor to have been involved with any one of the four. To be involved with all of them is beyond any expectations.

Many assisted with the collection of materials and with organizing and writing this book, especially Stu Kingma, M. I. D. Sharma, Frances Porcher, and Ann Mather. I am grateful to Mark Rosenberg for his help and his persistence in urging me to complete the manuscript, and to Sam Verhovek, Don Hopkins, and Dan Fox for their reviews and suggestions. Polly Hogan gave invaluable assistance in turning numbers into graphs, concepts into maps, and ideas into written text.

Ordering the material into a logical sequence with understandable sentences was the special contribution of Carolyn Bond, whose own experience living in India enriched her grasp of the material at hand. At the University of California Press, Lynne Withey, Hannah Love, Jacqueline Volin, and Sue Carter provided valuable ideas and guidance throughout the manuscript preparation process.

I also want to acknowledge countless mentors and friends, some mentioned in the book, and some mentioned, as it were, only in my mind. Truly, the book's coauthor is my wife, Paula. For over fifty years she has played a key part in my engagement in global health interests, and as I wrote these chapters, she not only compensated for my failing eyesight but also shared her acute sense for where the real story lay. When you are writing, it's often difficult to discern the wheat from the chaff; I thank Paula for her unerring instinct about what to leave in, and what to take out—as well as for her excellent suggestion for the book's title. To David, Michael, and Robert, I give heartfelt thanks for your sacrifices over the years.

PART ONE Africa

IDENTIFYING THE KEY STRATEGY

ONE A Loathsome Disease

You can smell smallpox before you enter the patient's room, but it's hard to describe. Even medical textbooks fall short when it comes to smells. The odor, probably the result of decaying flesh from pustules, is reminiscent of the smell of a dead animal. On at least two occasions, smell alone alerted me to the presence of smallpox. As I walked down a hospital hallway in India, the dead-animal odor stopped me in my tracks; following the smell, I located a smallpox patient. Another time, as I walked down an alley in an urban slum in Pakistan, the same smell hit me. There are competing smells in such places, but again one smell stood out. Knocking on doors, I found two siblings with smallpox.

Today, thirty years after the last recorded case of smallpox on the planet, I still find myself contemplating alternative tactics for its eradication, including one using smell. What if back then we'd been able to use trained dogs to identify smallpox patients? This would have sped up the searches in urban alleyways and railway stations, where people often lay on the ground, obscured under blankets.

Those of us working in the worldwide smallpox eradication program in the 1960s and 1970s made countless visits to smallpox patients. Most of these visits were to small, crowded, airless, single-room dwellings with the windows covered. In the dark, we were taken to the patient's bed, and it was possible, with a penlight, to examine the lesions and estimate the stage of the disease. Early on, the pocks would be surprisingly hard and deep. As the disease developed, they would fill with pus and soften, becoming pustules. Once the pustules began to break down, the mixture of pus and blood would stain the patient's bed and clothing. The person in the bed might have been happy and productive the previous week, but now had limited prospects of even seeing another day.

The disease took each of its hosts by surprise. They were not aware that a virus had entered their body and was silently establishing a beachhead by multiplying in the mindless way that viruses do. The virus carried no ill will; it was simply responding to the drive to perpetuate itself. It cannot reproduce on its own; it has to borrow cells from a human being. The borrowed cells put out ever more viruses, which in turn take over other cells.

Having borrowed and destroyed the cells in order to reproduce, the virus shows its gratitude, as it were, by wreaking havoc on its host. After two weeks of multiplication, just when the immune system is organizing a defense, the virus's host for the first time realizes something is wrong—a fever, a headache, perhaps a backache and vomiting. We all experience such symptoms occasionally, so the host doesn't worry. But after another two days, there is no denying the truth. The throat is sore because of lesions on the mucous membranes, and red bumps have appeared on the skin, especially on the face, arms, and legs. Over the next few days, the bumps turn to pustules. A robust immune system and a strong constitution might, at this point, turn the tide against the virus, and the host will recover. Even so, for most survivors, the price is high: pockmarks or even permanent blindness. Many, however, are unable to develop sufficient defenses; they die.

We saw some patients who didn't live long enough to develop pustules. The skin became swollen, the fever was high, and the patient became toxic. The virus completely overwhelmed the immune system.

The patient began to bleed with a hemorrhagic version of the disease that led, mercifully, to an early death.

Once the virus had left the host's body in absolute chaos, it sought out a new host to repeat the process. To me, the process made no sense—what was the purpose? What was the meaning? But the reality of nature seems to be that some species provide no evident benefit to the community of living organisms.

While working in the smallpox eradication program, I visited many villages. In one house I might find a baby, face swollen, eyes closed, breathing hard, with exposed surfaces thick with raised, pus-filled blisters. In such cases I would have to admit that there was nothing to be done. The devastated parents were about to lose the child. The next house might reveal two children lying in the same bed. At first glance they might appear well nourished, though sick with smallpox. However, lifting the blanket would reveal that they were very thin and poorly nourished. Their swollen faces, for just a moment, concealed their starvation.

In another house a young man might be wearing only a loincloth, because he didn't want anything touching his face or limbs, which were covered with lesions. His legs were bloody. He was trying not to move, grimacing in pain when he did. Any touch caused the lesions to bleed. His face was contorted with pain; he wanted only to die.

Each patient was part of a family and a community, yet others could do little to help. There was—and is—no cure for smallpox, and in this sense each patient faced the disease largely unaided. Shift your perspective to a larger scale of place and time, and these individuals become statistics—markers of suffering, but not the real thing. Shift your perspective again and the numbers become changes inflicted on whole cultures, dynasties, and nations, their place in history forever altered by this microscopic organism.

SMALLPOX IN HISTORY

Until its eradication, smallpox accompanied humans and human cultures throughout recorded history. Lesions are apparent on Egyptian mummies dating from the second millennium B.C.E. In 1979, Dr. Donald

Hopkins—instrumental in smallpox eradication in Sierra Leone and later in India—was allowed to examine the upper half of the mummified remains of Ramses V, who died in 1157 B.C.E. of a disease characterized by a rash.[1] Hopkins concluded that the rash he observed was compatible with a diagnosis of smallpox, although attempts to identify a virus in detached pieces of skin were unsuccessful.[2]

Hopkins details how the virus propagated itself in human populations through the centuries following Ramses' time, especially in Asia, Africa, and Europe. It came to the Americas with the European explorers, missionaries, and traders, who reported death rates exceeding 50 percent and as high as 90 percent among some indigenous peoples. In one of the saddest chapters in human history, proud, competent, and powerful groups were destroyed as settlers, carrying the smallpox virus and other diseases, moved into their ancestral homelands. From the Eastern seaboard, settlers carried smallpox with them as they moved westward in the 1830s and 1840s. Smallpox also traveled northward from what is now Mexico. The Blackfoot, once the most feared among Native American tribes, were decimated by smallpox. And the disease had, by 1837, reduced the population of the Mandan Indians to 150.[3]

Smallpox played a significant role at key moments in U.S. history as well. In the early battles of the Revolutionary War, American troops were placed at a disadvantage because they, unlike the British, had not been immunized by means of variolation, a prevaccination method then widely practiced in England that uses the smallpox virus itself to immunize. A risky procedure at best, variolation carried much greater risk in low-density populations, where smallpox was a sporadic disease and thus immunity levels in the population were low. The low immunity levels meant that variolation itself could cause widespread outbreaks. During the Battle of Quebec, on December 31, 1775, the Americans outnumbered the British, yet they were unable to sustain their attack because so many were weakened by smallpox. The English prevailed, and Canada remained with England rather than becoming part of the future United States. On February 5, 1777, after more than a year of deliberation, General George Washington gave the order to variolate all American troops. It was a tough decision with high military and medical risks: if the British learned of the program, they could have attacked while the American troops were sick, and the variolation itself, though much safer than smallpox, still destined some troops to die. By the time the British became aware of the operation, however, the two armies' susceptibility to smallpox was close to equivalent. Variolating the troops may have been Washington's most important tactical decision in the pursuit of independence.[4]

Nearly a century later, smallpox would come close to impacting what some historians have described as a watershed moment in U.S. history, when "the United States" shifted from a plural noun to a singular noun: Abraham Lincoln's delivery of the Gettysburg Address on November 19, 1863.[5] Reporters at the time described President Lincoln as appearing "sad, mournful, almost haggard." When he left that night for Washington, he had a severe headache and was forced to lie down, and for the next two weeks he was confined. His doctor originally diagnosed the illness as "bilious fever," and when a rash appeared, he called it scarlatina. A consultant, Dr. van Bibber, was called in to examine Lincoln, and he diagnosed the president's condition as smallpox. How Lincoln contracted the disease is unclear, but it might have happened while he was visiting hospitalized Union Army troops in Washington two weeks earlier. Had his incubation period been only one day shorter, the Gettysburg Address might not have happened.[6]

The clinical picture has varied through history and across geography in part because of differences in the strains of smallpox: the highest consistent death rates occurred in Asia (30 to 40 percent), intermediate death rates in West and Central Africa (20 to 30 percent), and the lowest in South America and certain parts of East Africa, where deaths were rare. High death rates among populations where the virus had only recently been introduced, as cited earlier for the Americas, usually resulted from the population's not having had a chance to develop resistance over the centuries. Yet that may be only part of the reason, since even in Southeast Asia, despite many centuries of exposure, smallpox still killed about one-third of those who became sick. So virus type also had a strong influence on mortality. Personal characteristics, including nutrition and variations in immune systems, may also have contributed to how different individuals reacted to the same virus. Population density had an indirect influence on mortality by affecting the age groups attacked. In low-density populations, occurrences tended to be sporadic and to affect all age groups when the virus was introduced, whereas in high-density populations, the disease was more a disease of childhood and young adulthood. In general, death rates are higher in the very young and the very old; therefore, changes in the ages of cases can change the mortality results.

THE DREAM OF ERADICATING SMALLPOX

The dream of eradicating smallpox had its beginning on May 14, 1796, when Edward Jenner, a physician practicing in Berkeley, England, inoculated cowpox taken from the hand of Sara Nelmes, a milkmaid, into the arm of a young boy named James Phipps. Jenner's experiment was grounded in his keen observational abilities and unusual patience. He was aware that poets described the complexions of milkmaids as lovely, and at the urging of his mentor, John Hunter, he applied himself to the question of why that would be true. Milkmaids, he observed, rarely had smallpox scars. Indeed, he had heard a milkmaid claim that she was protected from smallpox because she had previously had cowpox. He became convinced that the milkmaids' smallpox protection resulted directly from the cowpox sores on their hands, acquired from sores on cows' udders. Cowpox, unlike smallpox, was a self-limiting event and of little consequence.

Jenner, like other scientists of that time, lacked any understanding of viruses, immunology, vaccines, or vaccinology. He thought of the use of cowpox to protect people from smallpox in terms of mimicking nature. After twelve years of careful observation and note-taking, Jenner performed his experiment on the young James Phipps. A few days later, Phipps developed a sore at the site where cowpox had been inserted. After a few weeks, Jenner exposed the boy to smallpox by inoculating him with material collected from the lesions of a smallpox patient, using the method of variolation. The boy remained healthy, confirming

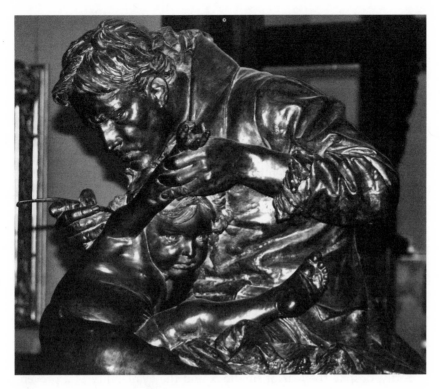

Figure 1. Statue of Edward Jenner vaccinating a child

what Jenner suspected: cowpox somehow provided protection against subsequent exposure to smallpox. In 1798, Jenner published an account of his experiment, a publication that has become a classic in the public health literature.[7] By attempting to copy nature, Jenner discovered the basic principle of vaccination. It is possible, using something similar to a deadly virus but itself innocuous, to fool a person's immune system into developing antibodies that destroy both viruses on contact. Over the years, scientists have made many vaccines by altering a virus that usually causes a disease. Vaccinologists have also learned how to modify the toxins caused by some organisms, such as the tetanus toxin, so that antibodies destroy the toxin itself. More recently, scientists have been working on vaccines against bacteria and, even more astounding, against parasites such as malaria. And viruses (with the exception of influenza) do not become immune to vaccines, as they do to antibiotics, so vaccines often provide lifelong protection. Jenner's discovery of this tool for preventing disease is one of the great breakthroughs in science. Indeed, the modern era of public health can be traced to Jenner's 1796 experiment.

Jenner saw the possibilities of his discovery and began to supply vaccine and instructions to interested persons. Thomas Jefferson, ever the scientist, also saw the potential and by 1801 had acquired vaccine from a medical friend in Boston. Jefferson personally administered the vaccine to his own household and to neighboring households around Monticello. Aware that Native Americans suffered from high smallpox death rates, he provided Meriwether Lewis and William Clark with vaccine to protect the tribes they met on their expedition across the continent between 1804 and 1806. This idea was better in theory than in practice, since they lacked a way of keeping the vaccine viable for long periods. In a letter to Jenner in 1806, Jefferson envisioned the eradication of smallpox: "Future nations will know by history only that the loathsome smallpox has existed."[8]

Sadly, despite the fear of smallpox and the availability of a preventive vaccine, effective vaccination programs were slow in coming and smallpox continued to be a scourge to the world. It was not until the middle of the twentieth century that the world began to fulfill the promise of Jenner's discovery and Thomas Jefferson's prediction. In 1958, the World Health Assembly (WHA), the governing body of the World Health Organization (WHO), passed a resolution to eradicate smallpox globally, and finally, in 1966, the WHA ratified a plan and a budget to support a global smallpox eradication program.

There are several reasons why the world had to wait 170 years after Jenner's work for smallpox to be eradicated. First, it was not until the 1960s that a vaccine was developed that could be produced in the countries where smallpox was endemic. Second, better vaccination techniques were developed, specifically, the jet injector, which was used in Africa and elsewhere around the world, and the bifurcated needle, which was tested in field trials and used widely, especially in India and Bangladesh.

Third, the new world order that emerged after World War II, including the development of the United Nations and WHO, made a global initiative possible. Fourth, enough people believed that eradication was possible. It took a new passion to proclaim that a disease that had plagued humanity for so long was not a fixed entity in the human landscape.

Finally, there was a crucial shift in vaccination strategy, from mass vaccination as the primary strategy to a highly focused form of surveillance and containment that turned out to be ideal for interrupting the progress of the smallpox virus. Surveillance and containment was envisioned from the beginning as the logical next step after mass vaccination had reduced the level of smallpox transmission; but it was found that surveillance and containment could be used as the primary strategy, speeding up the eradication effort. It was applied first in Nigeria in 1966 and 1967, then in other parts of West and Central Africa, and eventually elsewhere. It was refined six years later in the most intense smallpox area of the world: Bangladesh and the northern Indian states of Uttar Pradesh and Bihar. The chapters that follow track the story of this development.

TWO A Succession of Mentors

My participation in the smallpox eradication program was the result of my engagement with a host of mentors, some of whom I encountered only in books. Family, friends, and teachers also had a tremendous influence on me, the earliest, of course, being family.

My father was a Lutheran minister who was raised on a farm in Iowa. Growing up with four sisters and a brother in a series of parsonages provided me with an unvarnished, down-to-earth beginning in life. The houses always seemed too small. Each paycheck was cashed, and the money was distributed into Band-Aid cans marked for groceries, clothes, gas, and so on. My mother made many of the family's shirts and dresses, and clothes were handed down from one sibling to the next. A large garden, chickens, and one or two milk cows provided a major portion of the family diet. We canned food for the winter. The town's grocer—in Eldorado, Iowa (population one hundred)—always treated the family to a pint of ice cream when the grocery bill was paid at the end of each month.

When my family moved away from Eldorado, the town's population diminished by 8 percent. My father had received a call to a new church in Chewelah, Washington, a town of fifteen hundred people sixty miles north of Spokane. At the time, I thought Chewelah was a really big city. It was only when we moved twenty miles farther north, to Colville, that I realized what a big city was: Colville's population topped four thousand. There, my father started a new church.

Wherever we lived, my brother, four sisters, and I always had chores to do, and older siblings were responsible for supervising younger siblings. We were all expected to work hard but also to have fun, and we enjoyed much laughter and warmth. Games were a constant, even though some of the more conservative church members frowned upon such worldly frivolities. When the doorbell rang, playing cards would disappear in a flash, magically reappearing as soon as the visitor left. Our house was always intensely busy but well organized, and at the end of the day we children fell asleep to the comforting sounds of our mother playing hymns or classical music on the piano or violin, after which she often worked on correspondence courses.

My mother was not only well organized and interested in everything; she was also quite resourceful. Soon after my parents married in 1928, their Model T broke down a mile from home. Having grown up on a farm, my father was comfortable with mechanical repairs, and he set to work, asking my mother if she would walk home to fetch the pliers he needed to finish the job. His bride readily agreed but, having been raised in a city, she had no idea what pliers were and was too embarrassed to say so. By the time she arrived home she had a plan: she looked up "pliers" in the Sears catalog.

On another occasion, an ice storm brought below-freezing temperatures and took down the power lines. My father was away at a conference, and the hundreds of baby chicks in the chicken house, where lightbulbs warmed the interior to springlike temperatures, were at risk. My mother spread newspaper on the kitchen floor, closed the kitchen doors, let the chicks loose in the kitchen, and used the gas cooking stove to heat the room until the electricity was restored. The chicks survived. For a person who believed that cleanliness was next to godliness and who knew the smells of a chicken coop, this was an impressive approach to problem solving.

My father never let go of the work ethic he had learned growing up. He was always busy, calling on church members, visiting the sick in hospitals, or working in his study on his sermons and Sunday school lessons. He also tended the garden and the cows, helped with canning and house maintenance, and drove us children to music lessons or to work. He seemed content with his life choices, though when he was in his nineties he told me that he regretted that as a boy, he had never learned how to play, and that as a father, he had not played with us more when we were young.

My parents placed a high value on education. As children, all six of us were expected to take piano lessons and learn to play one other musical instrument, and it was assumed that we would go to college. Both at home and at our one-room school, there was little emphasis on science. Two of the first people to stir my interest in science were Shirley and Jim Kohlstedt. The Kohlstedts were just out of college, starting their own drugstore in Colville, living above the store. They later told me they hadn't really needed another employee, especially a thirteen-year-old who had just moved to town, but they were moved to sympathy by my apparent handicap. Having broken my leg during a basketball game, I had on a long leg cast, which was hidden by my trousers. When the cast was removed some weeks later and I walked into the store without a limp, they realized their mistake, but retained me as an employee anyway.

The Kohlstedts gave me a hands-on introduction to the world of science. Drugs altered the outcomes of disease, the metric system was an alternate way of measuring the world, and precision rather than opinion dictated how prescriptions were filled. Under their supervision, I filled prescriptions, demonstrating by oral test that I knew what each drug was intended to do. Soon I was also babysitting for their children and sharing in their family activities. I would come to realize that the best mentors not only have qualities one wants to emulate but also take a personal interest that often leads to involvement with their families and a relationship that continues through the years.

Tony Steiger, a frequent visitor at the drugstore soda counter, would become for me the epitome of a scientist. He was not a physically imposing man, but he was possessed of a keen intelligence and wide-ranging curiosity. He worked as an assayer, analyzing ore samples brought in by miners, but his interests went far beyond his work. He encouraged my budding interest in science, introducing me to the mysteries of logarithms. He taught me at night, in his home, and after each lesson I would experience the heady feeling that I knew a little more of a new and rarefied language.

When I was fifteen, I spent three months imprisoned in a body cast to treat a separation of the head of my femur. This was before the days of television in our town, which meant that I spent long hours reading, both for school and for pleasure. Albert Schweitzer's *Out of My Life and Thought* provided a glimpse into as foreign a world as I could imagine and left a lasting curiosity about other lands and peoples, the conditions of their lives and their health. I was hooked. I had earlier developed an interest in psychiatry as the result of reading a single novel about a colorful psychiatrist, but tropical medicine now became a competing interest. While in high school, I began subscribing to publications in both fields.

For two summers I worked for the U.S. Forest Service in Washington State and Oregon, and was regularly diverted to fight fires. The principles were simple and drilled into us repeatedly: separate the fuel from the flames, and the fire stops. Usually this meant building a fire line that went right down to soil so the flames could not cross it. At least two people would be sent to a fire, even a small one. We planned our approach with aerial maps and then carried in food and drinking water, basic firefighting tools, and lightweight sleeping bags made of paper. Water was almost never available to douse the fire. Our basic tool was a Pulaski, a combination ax and mattock that made it possible to cut down trees, chop logs in two, and dig a fire trench all with the same tool. Working in shifts, we would contain the fire as quickly as possible, hike back to the vehicle, report in, and be directed to the next fire. We might keep going for several days and nights in a row. During my second summer of firefighting, I graduated to chainsaw operator, with the task of determining the fire line's placement and cutting and removing logs that crossed the line. A series of Pulaski-wielding line builders would follow in leapfrog fashion, building the fire line as fast as the chainsaw operator could walk. Teamwork was essential—another valuable lesson I learned early in life.

TOWARD A CAREER IN EPIDEMIOLOGY

In 1953, I entered Pacific Lutheran University in Tacoma, Washington, as a biology major, which brought me into the sphere of influence of Bill Strunk, a charismatic biologist. He was tall with a full head of white, wavy hair that made me think of Einstein. He engendered great loyalty from young, impressionable, and eager students. A formidable instructor, he would walk from his office and down the corridor, his lecture already under way, to the classroom, where he would walk up to the blackboard and, without a pause, begin writing out phyla, families, classes, and genera with both hands simultaneously—an ability I have never again encountered. Strunk was my advisor when I applied to medical school at the University of Washington. A true scientist, if he was to recommend a student, he required the student to take a series of tests, including IQ tests, psychological tests, and tests of reasoning ability. If the student passed, Strunk became an active part of the process, mentoring the student right through admission and then maintaining contact over the years.

Before beginning my senior year at Pacific Lutheran, a classmate and I decided to arrive a week early to attend freshman orientation, so we could meet the new freshman girls before the other upperclassmen had a chance to. The plan worked better than I could have imagined. On Thursday evening of that week, as we sat outside the cafeteria after dinner, my friend offered me a challenge: "I will bet you a quarter you can't get a date with the next girl out of the door." A minute later, the door opened and out into the refreshing September evening walked Paula Ristad, a freshman from Palo Alto, California. She did not make it easy for me to win the bet. Having met me briefly at a freshman party earlier that week, she pegged me as a freshman. My attempt to impress her by saying I was a senior backfired. She concluded that I was both a freshman and a liar. My tenacity, however, eventually paid off. I started medical school at the University of Washington in 1957; Paula and I were married in December 1958. After our marriage, Paula transferred to the University of Washington to complete her degree in education.

In medical school, it was my good fortune to meet Rei Ravenholt, an epidemiologist who continued the chain of larger-than-life, charismatic people who influenced me. He had a booming voice and take-charge attitude that attracted students but also got him into disputes with peers. I was present the day he won a bet with some cancer researchers who had organized a study specifically to disprove Ravenholt's assertion that cancer is simply an extension of Darwin's law of evolution.[1] The study failed to disprove the assertion, and Ravenholt won the bet.

Besides teaching at the medical school, Ravenholt was also the Seattle–King County epidemiologist. Along with other medical students, I worked for him at the county health department after school, on Saturdays, and for several summers. Under Ravenholt's influence, public health became my primary interest, alongside my existing interest in tropical medicine, while my old interest in psychiatry faded. Public health and tropical medicine together pointed me in the direction of the relatively new field of global health, which is public health on a worldwide scale. At the time, global health was poorly defined, but I found it compelling .

Public health looks at illness and other risk factors in aggregate populations and comes up with wholesale solutions, such as changing the environment through water improvement or changing the resistance of the population to a certain disease through a mass immunization campaign. Its philosophical base is social justice, and its scientific base is epidemiology.

The first department of epidemiology in this country was established at Johns Hopkins School of Hygiene and Public Health in 1919. Wade Hampton Frost, who had received high praise for his studies on the 1918 influenza epidemic, was detailed by the U.S. Public Health Service to Johns Hopkins as the first resident lecturer. He later became a professor of epidemiology. Frost was a pioneer in epidemiology, originating the concept of the "index case," or first known case in an outbreak. Once the first case in an outbreak is identified, epidemiologists can work backward to determine the source of infection for that case and therefore for the entire outbreak.

Dr. Alex Langmuir, a graduate of Johns Hopkins, once summed up epidemiology as the selection of a numerator and a denominator to get a rate, and the gathering of enough information to interpret that rate. Clinical medicine concentrates on numerators, on the portion of society suffering from illness and seeking cure. Epidemiology addresses both numerators and denominators as it studies the distribution of illness or other conditions in the population as a whole.

In 1949, Langmuir began working at what was then called the Communicable Disease Center (CDC) in Atlanta, Georgia.[2] There, he developed the Epidemic Intelligence Service (EIS).[3] The original purpose of the EIS was to defend against possible biological warfare. The immediate source of the fear of biological attack was the unfounded belief that Korean hemorrhagic fever, which plagued both sides during the Korean War, had been intentionally introduced by the Chinese. (True to the Cold War spirit, the director of a viral research program in China told me in 1978 that his program had been started in response to the belief that the United States had intentionally brought Korean hemorrhagic fever into Korea.)

The practical training of the EIS epidemiologists for biological warfare can't wait for the real thing, so they focus on the everyday problems of public health in the United States and worldwide. The program helped to strengthen epidemiology as an integral part of public health practice. Langmuir had great confidence both in his own abilities and in the power of epidemiology to provide insight into how to prevent public health problems.

In 1962, after completing medical school and then an internship in New York, I joined the EIS training program at the CDC. Originally, I had intended to do an internal medicine residency in order to broaden my clinical background. Again, a mentor would influence the course of my life. Rei Ravenholt, visiting us in New York, was passionate about promoting epidemiology as a career specialty. He had been one of the first EIS officers, and he recommended that I apply to the EIS. I did, and was accepted. Instead of doing the residency, I headed for Atlanta.

THE THREAT OF SMALLPOX IN NEW MEXICO

In 1962, I became an EIS officer—a medical detective—and was stationed in Colorado. Paula and I made the drive from Atlanta to Denver during the final weeks of her pregnancy with our first son, David. She began having what threatened to be labor pains during the three-day trip. Our first stop in Denver was to make an appointment with an obstetrician at the Fitzsimmons Army Hospital, and the second stop was to get a motel room. We were still living in the motel when the real labor pains started and David was born. He spent his first week sleeping in a dresser drawer in the motel.

The assignment was exciting from the beginning. Within a month I had worked on a case of imported malaria, an outbreak of typhoid traced to a typhoid carrier in the southern part of the state, the introduction of the new Sabin oral polio vaccine, and several outbreaks of hepatitis. Seven months into my new position, I got a call from Drs. Don Millar and D. A. Henderson at the CDC. There was a suspected case of smallpox in Farmington, and they wanted me to check it out.

They told me that on Tuesday afternoon, March 19, 1963, a Dr. Frank Nordstrom, a pediatrician from Farmington, had called the CDC to report that a ten-month-old Navajo girl from a reservation, now hospitalized in Farmington, had a puzzling, vesicular rash. Nordstrom knew a great deal about rashes in children, but this one was different. He was concerned that it might be smallpox.

Millar and Henderson suggested that in the hours before my flight to Farmington I acquire *Smallpox*, a textbook written by C. W. Dixon.[4] The University of Colorado Medical School library had the book, but it was checked out to a student. First, I had to find the student. Second, I had to convince him that my need was greater than his—no mean feat, as he was writing a paper. I succeeded in talking him out of the book and then read key sections of it at the airport and during the flight. As the plane came to a stop on the Farmington airport tarmac that evening, I felt relatively comfortable with my knowledge about the clinical differences between smallpox and other diseases, especially chickenpox. I was unnerved when I saw the car waiting at the foot of the airplane stairs.

The local health department staff whisked me to the hospital, where a group was waiting for the diagnosis by the out-of-town expert—a twenty-seven-year-old EIS officer who had never seen a case of smallpox.

Scrubbed and gowned, I entered the patient's room. It was only a few steps from the door to the bed, hardly enough time to consider every diagnostic possibility, but my comfort in understanding the differential diagnosis crumbled in those few steps. I saw a very sick, lethargic, feverish baby. Her young mother hovered nervously as I examined the girl. The lesions, primarily on her extremities, were round, single-chambered, and well circumscribed, yet they were not typical of either smallpox or chickenpox. After sending specimens off to the CDC, I phoned Henderson and Millar in Atlanta to review the findings. Since we did not yet know what was going on, we had to treat the situation as "possible smallpox" until the laboratory results were returned.

If this was smallpox, it was a very big public health event. The last case of smallpox in the United States, in 1949, was the result of an importation of the disease to New York. Many still remembered the hundreds of people in lines snaking around city blocks waiting to get vaccinated. The working definition of an "outbreak" is "an unusual occurrence" of a disease. The definition is thus situational, different for different diseases, and even different for the same disease depending on geography. For many infectious diseases, dozens or even hundreds of cases might be required for it to be called an outbreak. For smallpox in the United States, a single case would qualify as an outbreak.

The state and local health departments in New Mexico made staff and vehicles available, and we launched an immediate effort to do several things simultaneously. First, we needed to track the child's contact with other people for the previous three weeks, even secondary contacts, and determine their histories of recent illness. Second, we had to learn about outsiders who might have come to the area and about trips by local persons to other parts of the world, even in the absence of evidence of direct contact with the child. An undetected case of smallpox, or even two generations of the disease, could have occurred between the introduced case and the current case. Third, we had to identify every person who had been in contact with the child who could be at risk if this proved to

be smallpox. Finally, we needed to begin a vaccination program immediately for everyone with potential contact with the child to prevent
secondary cases. Vaccination even days after exposure can still prevent
the disease or modify its severity.

After initiating these efforts, I spent the remainder of the first full day
on the Navajo reservation, reconstructing time lines, questioning people,
and vaccinating contacts. That night I learned that the initial laboratory report results were compatible with smallpox. The seriousness of
the situation was increasing. Late that night I read a local newspaper
interview with a former medical missionary who had worked in Asia
and was familiar with smallpox. He had seen the hospitalized child and
thought her symptoms were typical of smallpox.

Dr. Nordstrom, the child's pediatrician, had me stay at his house,
so concerned was he that I have nothing else to worry about. The next
morning, on the drive to the hospital, he took a long, scenic route, saying
that he did so every morning to get "centered" before meeting the problems of the day. It struck me as an important mental health prescription
for anyone, and especially for people in his line of work.

Over the next several days we established that tourists from Asia
had recently come to Farmington, but they had no connection, even
indirectly, with the child. Men from the reservation had been to Mexico,
but none reported exposure to anyone with a rash disease.

Control procedures were superb. Every possible contact was found
and vaccinated, and the child remained in isolation. She was improving
clinically, and her mother began to relax. On the third day, two pieces
of information ended the control efforts. We had mapped the lesions
daily; now, new lesions had developed that were not typical of smallpox.
Smallpox starts with red bumps, progresses to vesicles (blisters), then to
pustules, and finally to scabs. The progression is consistent in any one
area of the body, though it may be at different stages in different areas.
Now we were seeing new bumps in areas that had already progressed
through blisters and scabbing. Then came the definitive CDC laboratory
report: the first report had been erroneous. It wasn't smallpox; it was
herpes virus.

What made the case so confusing? The child, in addition to having pneumonia, severe thrush, and enteritis, was recovering from measles, which had left a base rash on top of which were superimposed lesions of disseminated herpes. The child recovered well, the physician and the investigators breathed a sigh of relief, and life returned to normal. But it was a peripheral brush with what could have been a deadly disease.[5]

One month later, in April, I returned to Atlanta for the annual EIS conference, during which current officers had the opportunity to present cases to their peers and the CDC staff. The report of the smallpox scare naturally generated high interest. Many former officers found the week-long gatherings so stimulating that they would attend the conference on their own time and money just to hear about the latest investigations. The camaraderie among EIS officers tends to be lifelong. An annual publication updated information on the location of current and former EIS officers, and officers would often seek each other out in institutions or overseas locations.

At this meeting it was announced that the physician who served the Peace Corps volunteers in India had to leave his post unexpect-edly because of illness, and the Peace Corps was looking for a short-term replacement while they recruited his successor. The duties would include traveling throughout India to provide medical care for Peace Corps volunteers and arranging for ongoing care by local practitioners. Because of my interest in global health, I decided to volunteer. After interviews in Washington, D.C., I was accepted for the position, and after many briefings, I departed in May 1963 for a three-month tour of duty in India.

SEEING SMALLPOX IN INDIA

As is true for so many travelers to India, my first few hours in the coun-try were overwhelming. My flight landed at 3 A.M. in New Delhi. May is a very hot month in North India, and my initial reaction as I walked down the steps from the plane was disorientation: it could not possibly be this hot in the middle of the night. But it was. As I left the baggage area I stepped out into a virtual sea of people, many pressing in to be the one to take my suitcase and briefcase, escort me to a vehicle, and deliver me to my next destination. With experience one becomes accustomed to this scene, but the first time is entirely confusing. Just in time, I saw a sign with my name on it held by the Peace Corps driver assigned to meet me. We drove to the hotel through predawn streets already crowded with people. By the time I checked in at my hotel, I had experienced two of the constants in India: heat and crowding.

Yet this was only a hint of what was to come. Summer temperatures that year reached 50 degrees Centigrade (122 degrees Fahrenheit). I saw asphalt roadways so soft that they retained the footprints of people crossing the street. A walk through Old Delhi's markets was an immersion in real crowding. Yet what I expected to be a totally overwhelming experience turned out to be surprising as I saw how people could be cheerful, resourceful, and productive in situations that would have left most Westerners demoralized and unable to function.

During this assignment I worked under the supervision of Dr. Charlie Houston and found in him yet another important mentor. He was a cardiologist by training and a mountain climber and social activist by avocation. He worked over the years trying to develop an artificial heart, and he became a world authority on high-altitude physiology. Houston was an example of undaunted courage and had long been famous in mountain-climbing circles for his role in an attempt, in 1953, to rescue a sick climber from K-2, the second-highest mountain on earth, during a storm.[6] He faced each day with the cheerful confidence that he could make a difference, and the challenges of doing health work in a developing country never seemed to dampen his enthusiasm.

Houston made sure that in addition to taking care of Peace Corps volunteers, I made rounds at hospitals so I could begin to understand the health problems facing India. This was my first opportunity to see smallpox patients. The experience was life changing. Textbook descriptions miss the often catatonic appearance of patients attempting to avoid movement, the smell of rotting pustules that permeates the room, and the social and psychological isolation imposed by the disease. I had seen polio patients in iron lungs who could see their families only through a window and with the help of a mirror. Smallpox separated patients from their loved ones, too, but in a different way. Pustules mixed with pus and blood might cover the face. The smell was overpowering. Visitors recoiled, and even hospital staff tried to avoid touching the patient.

And, since smallpox patients were getting no specific treatment, being in the hospital offered no medical advantage to them. It merely ensured quarantine. Even if patients recovered, they would likely have lifetime facial scars, in which case the social separation in the hospital was simply a harbinger of their future life. I left India with the conclusion that although many diseases and conditions are tragic, smallpox was in a class by itself for the misery it inflicted on both individuals and society.

A RESEARCH PROJECT IN TONGA

Nine months after returning to the United States from India, I said yes to another foreign assignment. D. A. Henderson asked me to go to Tonga as part of a CDC research team. The CDC had incorporated a new vaccination technology, the jet injector, into its programs, and the Tonga study was meant to determine if the smallpox vaccine could be effectively diluted for use in the jet injector, and if so, what the optimal dilution would be. Tonga had not had smallpox or a smallpox vaccination program since the early 1900s; therefore, it provided a virgin population in terms of smallpox antibodies. The plan was to use different dilutions of vaccine on different population groups, compare the results, and determine the optimal dilution.

The CDC research team arrived on the island of Tonga on Easter weekend of 1964. Dr. Ron Roberto was the team leader for a group that included Drs. Peter Greenwald and Pierce Gardner, as well as Vachel Blair, a movie photographer who would be making a documentary of the project titled *Miracle in Tonga*. The final leg of the trip was in a small plane from Nandi, Fiji, to Nuku'alofa, Tonga. We landed on a grass airstrip in a classic South Sea island paradise.

However, the sense of being in paradise was almost immediately shattered. We learned on arrival that a major earthquake had occurred in Alaska, and there was concern about a tidal wave spreading throughout the Pacific and ultimately coming to Tonga. The main island is quite flat, and the guesthouse where our team was supposed to stay was on the north end of the island. Our hosts decided that we should be driven to the south end of the island, for safety's sake.

As we settled into our temporary lodgings, we set up a schedule of two-hour shifts so that one person would remain awake listening to the radio, which was broadcasting emergency reports through the night in Tongan and English. About 2 A.M., the radio announcer reported that a tidal wave this far south had not materialized, so the station was going off the air until morning, as usual. The person listening decided to turn off the radio, let everyone continue sleeping, and explain what had happened in the morning. At 5 A.M., another member of the group woke up, turned on the radio, and found only static. Assuming the tidal wave had hit and knocked out the radio station, he woke the team as well as the people in the surrounding houses to alert them to the arrival of the (thankfully nonexistent) tidal wave. It was an exciting beginning to our stay.

The vaccine dilution testing project went well. We learned how to use and fix jet injectors, and by comparing various dilutions with a standard vaccination group we decided on a 50:1 dilution as optimal. The results of the study were very useful a few years later when the West and Central African smallpox eradication program used the jet injector to deliver measles vaccine to children and smallpox vaccine to the entire population. With this useful tool, tens of millions of injections were given within a few short years.

CAN SMALLPOX BE ERADICATED?

Earlier in 1964, before going to Tonga, I had read an article in the *New England Journal of Medicine* that prompted me to decide, on the spot, that I wanted to study with the author, Dr. Tom Weller.[7] Weller had presented the *Journal* article the previous year as the commencement address to the Harvard Medical School. He expressed a vision of global health that I wanted to explore. He was saying to those young graduates: now that you have developed these medical skills and the knowledge that goes with them, think about using them in the parts of the world that need them the most.

In the fall of 1964, I left my job as an EIS officer with the CDC to begin an academic year in the Tropical Public Health Department at Harvard, of which Weller was chair. During that year of study I had the opportunity to spend considerable time with Weller, a Nobel Prize–winning scientist.[8] I had gone to Harvard to study global health, not smallpox, but when it came time to choose a topic to present in Weller's spring semester seminar class, I decided to write a paper on the possibility of eradicating smallpox globally. At the time, I had no way of knowing that I would be involved in exactly such a venture by the following year.

The paper was a purely academic exploration of what might be involved. In India I had seen the absolute misery of smallpox patients. In Tonga I had seen that the jet injector offered a standardized vaccination method that could be used widely with reliable take rates (a "take" is a successful vaccination as evidenced by the appearance of a sore, crater, or blister at the vaccination site several days after the vaccination). The smallpox vaccine was good; it lasted ten years or more, and it was inexpensive. Moreover, the smallpox virus's life cycle did not involve a non-human host, which would have complicated the strategy (yellow fever eradication had failed when it was found that nonhuman primates also harbored the virus). And because of the disease's obvious symptoms, surveillance (tracking a disease) was relatively easy. Finally, people—including government officials—feared the disease and were therefore likely to cooperate. Citizens would likely participate, and governments would likely fund the program. I used the word *eradicate* in my presentation quite deliberately both because I believed in the possibility of eradication and because many people didn't. Some believed that eradication was impossible because of the failed attempts at eradicating both yellow fever and malaria. Others assumed that emptying a viral niche was impossible—even though species extinction occurs all the time.

My presentation sparked an intense debate. Weller's own questioning unnerved me at first. He probed from various angles, exposing the weakness of my arguments by using the failed attempts at malaria eradication as his lever. Later, one of his staff members told me that Weller would never deliberately embarrass a student and that his intense questioning was meant to explore ideas he thought had merit.

A classmate, Dr. Yemi Ademola, head of preventive medicine for Nigeria, continued the discussion with me for weeks after the seminar. He became so interested in the possibility of a smallpox eradication program in Nigeria that he eventually traveled to Atlanta to discuss its possibilities with D. A. Henderson and Alex Langmuir. They had already been working with WHO officials to secure a commitment from the World Health Assembly to adopt the global goal of smallpox eradication.[9]

Indeed, other people had been thinking along similar lines for some time. Several years before smallpox eradication was discussed at the CDC and WHO, Charlie Houston had suggested a program to eliminate smallpox from India by using Peace Corps volunteers to head up mobile vaccination teams. His plan was rejected at the time in Washington, D.C. Rei Ravenholt had a similar idea and wrote to Sargent Shriver, head of the Peace Corps, on June 24, 1961, suggesting that the Peace Corps launch a smallpox eradication program using Peace Corps volunteers to train vaccination teams, all supervised by medical officers. Ravenholt notes in his letter that there is "no technological obstacle to its rapid eradication."[10] A movement toward smallpox eradication seemed to be building from many directions.

THREE Practicing Public Health in Nigeria

The possibility of eradicating smallpox interested me, but since medical school, I had held a different vision of what my career would be. I wanted to do public health work in medical missions in developing countries.

It had always disturbed me that church groups did so much medical work in developing countries yet took so little responsibility for disease prevention. Mission boards rarely encouraged it, even though prevention is the most efficient use of limited resources. This of course made them little different from health care delivery systems in the United States. A June 1965 response I received from the Board of Foreign Missions of the United Lutheran Church of America was typical: "Our medical personnel are unable to do much in preventive medicine on a community scale. Understaffing and time limit what they can do in this area." The board had missed the point.[1] One possible explanation for this stance is that medical work had become such a useful proselytizing tool. Clinics and hospitals attract people and can leave them feeling indebted after they have received help. I always felt that was wrong. Churches should be working because of what they believe, not because of what they are trying to get other people to believe.

Prevention, on the other hand, often goes unappreciated. When people do not realize they might otherwise be susceptible to a disease, they feel no urge to thank someone for a vaccination or other preventive measure, much less adopt that person's religious beliefs. People rarely reflect on the fact that they have not had to deal with smallpox, tuberculosis, whooping cough, diphtheria, rabies, or other controlled maladies in their lifetimes. Yet this is not by chance. Every disease encounter missed is the result of deliberate actions taken by unknown benefactors in the past. It is one of the clear attractions of work in public health: the public health practitioner can remain anonymous.

I found an unexpected ally for my views, as well as a mentor, in Dr. Wolfgang Bulle, medical secretary for the Lutheran Church–Missouri Synod. Bulle had obtained his medical training in Germany during World War II, and he suffered from what seemed to be posttraumatic stress disorder, especially in relationship to his experiences on the Eastern Front as the Soviets moved into Germany. Perhaps out of a need to extirpate the images of those days, he worked for ten years as a surgeon in a mission hospital in South India. An unusually intense workaholic who abhorred wasting time, he seemed to work much of the night reading, underlining, and making notes. Certain there were better ways of addressing the health problems of the developing world than the traditional hospital-based approach, he was willing to try community prevention. With enthusiasm, he posted our family of three—Paula, our three-year-old son, David, and myself—to the Ogoja area of Eastern Nigeria, where a clinic was being set up in the small town of Yahe. Neither Bulle nor I knew exactly what I would be doing. The idea was to go there, learn the language and culture, and see what the needs were. We did have a clear picture of the goal, however: to integrate community-based prevention into a church health program.

VILLAGE LIFE IN NIGERIA

In August 1965, Paula, David, and I took the *Queen Elizabeth* to South-ampton, spent ten days at the London School of Hygiene and Tropical Medicine getting advice on leprosy, tuberculosis, and African health conditions, and then sailed from Liverpool to West Africa on an Elder Dempster Line ship, which allowed us some time to acclimate to the temperature and to read up on our new home as we traveled south. We disembarked at Lagos, at that time the capital of Nigeria. Lagos was hot, humid, colorful, noisy—and crowded. People were accustomed to mov-ing in very close quarters, whether on the street, in queues, in taxi cabs, or in the market. My brief experience in India was somewhat of a prepa-ration, but this was all new for Paula and of course David. After several days in Lagos, we traveled to Nigeria's Eastern Region, stopping for a night in the city of Enugu, the region's capital. Though much smaller than Lagos, Enugu nevertheless offered shopping and amenities that, on occasion during the coming months, would lure us into making the three-hour drive from our village home ninety miles northeast, over dirt roads that seemed to test our body parts' ability to remain connected.

Dr. Bulle had arranged for us to spend our first six months in the village of Okpoma, about fifteen miles from Yahe, so we could learn the local language, Yala, and learn about the culture through daily con-tact with the villagers. Our home in Okpoma was a mud-walled house with four rooms: a living room, a kitchen, a "master" bedroom, and a bedroom for David. There was no electricity, running water, or indoor bathroom. For washing up, we put a tub on the floor of David's room and carried in water. In the village, the living room of every home was considered communal. It was not only accepted but expected that village members would enter our living room and sit down to observe and learn about us. This they did daily, so the learning was reciprocal.

The village was far quieter than the cities, except at night. Every night resounded with drumming. An important chief from our village had died just before our arrival, so drumming occurred nightly for the first several weeks. We quickly became accustomed to the noise and found that it actually provided a soothing background to sleep.

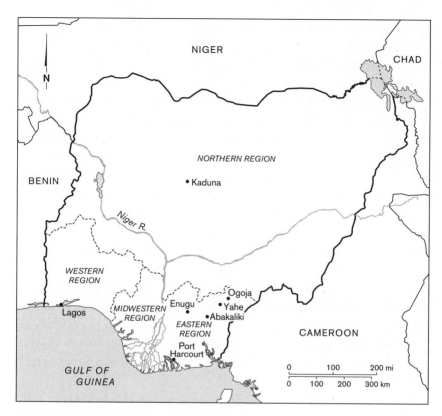

Map 1. Nigeria, 1966–67

We had been instructed on how to behave when the current village chief made his first visit, including offering him a glass of palm wine. We also were informed that he much preferred beer. One day soon after we arrived the chief came to the house, sat in our living room, and conversed with us through an interpreter. When we offered him a glass of beer, he was obviously pleased. The custom with palm wine was to sip off the top layer of the liquid, which could contain foreign material and insects, and spit that mouthful out before consuming the wine itself. Following that practice, he sipped the beer's top layer and, to our surprise, spit it on the living room wall. Our three-year-old son was obviously impressed. That night, before going to bed, he asked for a glass of powdered milk. He took a mouthful and spit it on the wall!

It was September when we arrived, shortly before the rainy season yielded to the dry season. As the dry season progressed, we came to appreciate the sheer luxury of year-round water available at the tap at home in the States. The village's name, "Okpoma," means "place of the salt." The ground contained so much salt that it provided a commercial industry for local inhabitants. However, the well water was too saline for consumption. Water catchments were used during the rainy season. In the dry season, the villagers would walk to streams and water holes to get drinking water. As the hot, dry weather continued and nearby water sources dried up, they had to travel longer and longer distances on foot to access larger water sources. This work most often fell to the women.

Life was not easy for any of the villagers; however, the women worked incredibly hard, while the men could often be seen resting. During the dry season, the women's day would start early with a three- to five-mile walk to a water source; the women would return with heavy pots of water balanced on their heads. Two morning water trips were followed by work in the yam fields, and finally a trip late in the day for firewood to prepare the evening meal.

We gradually learned how to bargain. A market was held every fifth day in our village, and markets were held in other villages on a preordained circuit during the other four days. Markets would provide the usual local foods, clothing, flashlights, kerosene, matches, and so on. As part of the market, or on separate days, there would be opportunities to buy fresh beef. Small herds of cattle would be driven from northern Nigeria by young men and boys, usually from the Fulani tribe, and a local entrepreneur would buy a cow and butcher it for sale. The price was 2 shillings (0.28 cents) a pound, regardless of cut, and the entire animal would be sold within hours. Because of the long walks experienced by the cattle, the meat, no matter which cut, was sufficiently tough that it required cooking in a pressure cooker. For most other things, bargaining was required. Initially, after thinking a fair deal had been concluded, we would find that we had endangered the local economy by paying far too much.

At our house, we hired a young man to bicycle to the closest water source during the dry season with two ten-gallon tins tied on his bike rack. When full, the two tins weighed about 160 pounds. By the end of the dry season, when the water trips were long, he could make no more than two daily trips, but this provided adequate water for our small household. Boiling the drinking water on the propane stove took hours every day. The boiled water was stored in bottles in a kerosene refrigerator, which also put out heat, increasing the temperature in the house to even more uncomfortable levels. In late November the annual *harmattan*, the breeze from the north, arrived—a welcome event because it cooled off the temperatures even though it brought sand and dust from the Sahara Desert, dimming the sun and leaving everything dark and gritty. A dusted table would be covered with another layer of dust within an hour. Mosquito nets on the beds—necessary to reduce the chance of catching malaria—kept out not only mosquitoes and rodents but also any welcome breeze that might have come through the room at night. During the hottest months we sometimes sat up for hours at night to avoid getting into a stifling bed.

We had read about the arrival of the first rains, which usually occurs in March, but to experience the relief they brought was something else again. The water poured down in torrents. People left their houses and gathered in the rain, dancing and rejoicing. The rains signaled the end of the dry season and promised new crops, cooler temperatures, and the end of the long trips for water.

To practice community health in another culture requires an understanding and appreciation of that culture. But it's also arrogant to assume you can truly understand it. Paula and I had daily lessons in Yala from an American who had settled in the area six months before us and who was the first foreigner to analyze the language. We learned to prepare local foods with pounded yams and cassava, and to bargain in the markets, which were held according to the local five-day calendar. The calendar had existed for as long as anyone could remember, and was still used alongside the seven-day weekly calendar introduced by the British.

As much as we learned, the differences between the villagers' experience and ours always remained starkly evident. For one thing, we could leave any time we wanted. For another, we had access to basic health knowledge and the money to be able to apply it, while the villagers did not. To cite just one example, we arrived in the village at the end of a whooping cough epidemic. The characteristic coughs, or whoops, which often go on for weeks, persisted throughout the village at night during our early weeks in the village, making clear the price paid for not having routine childhood immunizations. We were able to provide our child not only with immunizations but also with prophylaxis against malaria, screened windows to protect against mosquitoes, bed nets, and safe water. The villagers could not do this for their children. They did not have access to such basic health practices. They had to spend the little money they had, the equivalent of $1 per day, on food and shelter.

While village life in Africa offered a predictable rhythm and the benefits of community, I was also struck by its limitations. People with wealth and education in a country like the United States can read about a new idea in the *New York Times* in the morning and be applying it in the afternoon. Those without education or money, whether in the United States or in Africa, cannot. Lacking the resources to change their future, they fall prey to a certain fatalism. Through the years I have come to see fatalism, the assumption that you can't really change your future, as one of the great challenges in global public health.

Another lesson I have learned over time is to respect culture as a powerful force; when you tangle with it, culture always wins. Thus, it's essential to approach any culture and its customs with respect. An early demonstration of the power of culture occurred one evening in Okpoma. Some neighbors were visiting us in our courtyard. One of the women had been stung by a scorpion—a very painful condition but usually not fatal for adults. I offered her the usual medical treatment, an injection of a local anesthetic. She refused and instead wanted to see the local healer. We walked to his house and watched as he spit into the dirt to make a paste and applied it to her sting. From the standpoint of Western medicine, this treatment could have brought no immediate medical benefit, yet she immediately stopped crying and moaning. It was a dramatic example of the power of belief in the effectiveness of a traditional cultural practice.

While contact with other expatriates was limited, I did find a men-

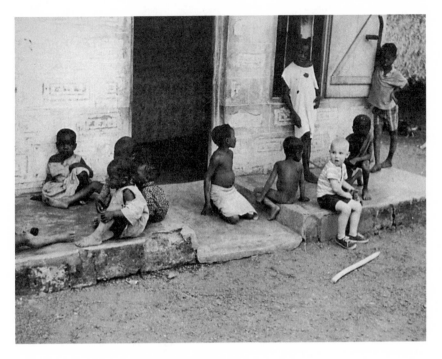

Figure 2. David Foege and village children, Nigeria, 1965

tor in Nigeria—another former EIS officer, Dr. Herman Gray, who was doing missionary work. Paula, David, and I spent a weekend with him. Besides sharing many observations about diseases and their treatment under African conditions, Gray gave us a primer on snake bites. He had a collection of preserved snakes that he used as a reference to identify the dead snakes that people brought to him when they sought treatment for snake bite. The people's well-justified fear of snakes made it even more astounding that they could find the courage to walk barefoot on paths after dark. We saw this fear demonstrated when our house-helper, Lawrence Atutu Ochelebe, on finding a snake in our house, beat not only the snake but also the broom into an unrecognizable pulp.

After six months, Paula, David, and I moved to the medical compound at Yahe, and I began working in the clinic. In Yahe we still lacked electricity but did gain the luxuries of running water and a bathroom. Here I joined three nurses in running clinics while putting my new language skills to use. In rural Africa, where separate languages coexisted in small geographic areas, learning one local language was only a beginning. At the clinic we might see patients from more than twenty different language groups in the course of a week. Sometimes three interpreters were required to communicate with a single patient, increasing the opportunity for errors of interpretation.

The combination of pathogens we would see in a single child was often a source of dismay. A young girl might appear at the clinic with a case of measles, but an examination would then disclose that she was also malnourished. She might also have malaria parasites circulating in her blood, microfilaria from onchocerciasis coursing through her body, blood in her urine because of schistosomiasis, and hookworms, roundworms, and whipworms in her intestine. Most of these problems could have been avoided by simple measures, such as wearing shoes, using bed nets, and drinking safe water.

AN INVITATION FROM THE CDC

By March 1966, my family and I had settled into the work of the clinic and life in Yahe. I was making plans for the community work that was most needed—improving water supplies, improving childhood nutrition, and setting up immunization programs—when an unexpected letter arrived from the CDC. In February, the World Health Assembly (WHA) executive board had approved a global smallpox eradication effort, a plan that was sure to be passed at the WHA's annual meeting in May. The program would be administered by WHO with the assistance of the CDC. Could I be available as a consultant for setting up the program in the Eastern Region of Nigeria?

The CDC followed up by sending Dr. Henry Gelfand to Enugu to meet with me, explore my interest, and talk over the details of a contract. Henry was one of a handful of public health people assigned to work with the new smallpox eradication program at the CDC. The program was initially headed by D. A. Henderson; Don Millar took over when Henderson moved to WHO to head up its global program. Henry made it clear that he was skeptical about having an outside consultant on the team, who might have dual loyalties. He would have preferred a full-time CDC employee. I, on the other hand, was enthusiastic about being a consultant. I would be able to continue to do public health in Africa and pursue my interest in smallpox. I also saw the program's possible long-term benefits for developing immunization programs in Eastern Nigeria. An additional incentive was the news that an EIS colleague, Dr. Stan Foster, would be in charge of the CDC workers in Nigeria. During the EIS course at the CDC in 1962, because of alphabetical seating, Stan and I sat next to each other, and that was the beginning of a lifelong friendship. The Fosters were at home anywhere. Stan would prove tireless in his dedication to the concept of global health, first in Nigeria and years later in Bangladesh.

I accepted the invitation to attend the July training session for the first smallpox teams at the CDC in Atlanta. Because of my immediate experience in Nigeria, I was asked to lecture to the trainees on health conditions in West Africa. The timing of the trip to Atlanta was perfect for my family. Paula was now pregnant with our second son, Michael, and he could be delivered in the United States.

I assumed that consulting for the smallpox program in Eastern Nigeria would be a temporary diversion in a career dedicated to public health in Africa. In fact, it turned out to be a decisive shift in direction for my entire life's work.

THE EBB AND FLOW OF SMALLPOX

During my six months in Okpoma and subsequent months in Yahe, I had not seen any smallpox cases, but I knew that smallpox was a much-feared phenomenon in the area. In rural Africa smallpox was typically not a constant threat in a particular geographic area. Rather, it was a recurrent visitor, returning to an area after five, ten, or even twenty or more years, depending on the population and its degree of contact with other areas. While smallpox is tenacious in finding susceptible new victims and devastating in its effect, it is not as contagious as some infectious diseases. Although described as "a highly contagious viral disease" in some recent books, smallpox is in fact far less contagious than influenza or measles.[2] Household secondary attack rates for measles can be as high as 80 percent—that is, if a single person contracts measles, 80 percent of susceptible people in that person's household will become ill one generation later. For smallpox, the secondary attack rate might only be 30 percent. In Africa, measles outbreaks would often be recorded in a village every second or third year; transmission was so great that only a few susceptible children were needed to insure transmission. But a village might go decades between outbreaks of smallpox.

Smallpox transmission was typically lower during the rainy season, when humidity was higher and people traveled less. As travel increased again after the monsoons, the virus would also be on the move again through its human vectors. A village's residents would conclude, after some years without a smallpox case, that smallpox was a problem of the past, only to have the virus arrive with a visitor, vendor, traveler, or returning resident. The resulting outbreak would become the consuming event of the village as the virus slowly, over weeks and months, infected much of the cohort born since its last visit, plus some older villagers who had somehow escaped infection during the last outbreak.

The outbreak would totally destroy the rhythm of life, interfering with farming and commerce as the youngest parents were infected, often from their children, and as families buried the dead. The anthropologist Laura Bohannan, who was living with the Tiv people of Northern Nigeria when smallpox devastated the tranquil scene, described the outbreak in her novel *Return to Laughter*. The local people, she notes, called smallpox "water," and she soon came to understand the meaning. "By now I thought of smallpox as water," she writes, "as a treacherous hungry sea beating steadily against crumbling dikes. . . . At the first advance of the water, the countryside had seethed and boiled with the movement of people fleeing before it."[3]

She describes the resulting terror, death, and hate: "Fear crept shadow-like over their faces; it jerked at their gestures, sharpened their voices and sapped their hearts. . . . It marked us all and left the sign for others to read." She continues, "People held by the tenderest bond of love and affection could, when plague struck, leave each other to die in lonely terror. It must be thus when empires fall, and a whole society goes crashing into ruin. The fear that tears father from child, brother from brother, husband from wife. Where there is no law but nightmare. . . . But there is one thing greater than terror: fatigue. . . . There is nothing left in our minds, our hearts or nerves or bodies to show that we lived."[4] In the West, she says, the closest experience is the horror of war.

As the epidemic waned, the survivors realized they would carry the physical scars—pockmarks on the face, or even blindness—for life; in many cases, these vestiges of the disease interfered with marriage and social relationships. The outbreak became part of the village oral history, discussed less frequently and with less passion as months and years passed, until once again the collective memory dimmed and the village let down its guard. The interval between outbreaks might shorten because of increased population density, but this did not change the cycle of a village's thinking. The villagers would gradually forget about smallpox as time passed, only to face the shock of it again when it returned.

A recent review of smallpox in Africa helps clarify this ebb and flow of smallpox as recorded by the colonial powers in Africa in the late nineteenth and early twentieth centuries.[5] England, France, Portugal, and Belgium, after taking control of large areas of Africa following the Berlin Conference of 1884–85, introduced health services as part of developing their empires. One of the few tools they had to offer was smallpox vaccine, and they kept records on vaccinations given and known smallpox cases.

From 1928 to 1960, between fifteen and thirty thousand cases of smallpox were reported per year in Africa. However, given the paucity of clinics and hospitals and the unreliability of reporting, the true number was probably ten to one hundred times higher. Health officials welcomed the years of decline and blamed the subsequent increases on people's reluctance be vaccinated, on importations from other countries, or on variolation.[6]

THE PRACTICE OF VARIOLATION

Africa, like other parts of the Old World, especially India and China, had maintained a tradition of variolation as a tool for limiting, if not preventing, the full impact of smallpox when it struck. Variolation (also called inoculation) is often confused with vaccination. *Vaccination* refers to the transfer of virus material that is not smallpox but is similar enough to it that the person develops antibodies effective against the smallpox virus. *Variolation* is the much more ancient practice of transferring material from the pustule of a smallpox patient to the abraded skin of a healthy person. Variolation therefore involves transferring the smallpox virus itself, rather than a surrogate virus. There is still some risk of death. However, the mortality rates with variolation are much lower than when the virus is transmitted naturally, through the respiratory tract—perhaps 1 or 2 percent fatalities from variolation versus 20 to 30 percent from natural infection.

In most variolation practices, the virus is introduced through the skin. It is believed that in China, however, the intranasal route (insufflation) was used, with powdered scabs that had been stored for some time and that had been obtained from patients with few lesions. Presumably the low number of lesions indicated a less virulent virus and thus a less severe infection in the recipient. The practice may have developed independently in India, China, and Africa, although some believe that it originated in India and spread from there.[7]

Certainly one of the enduring mysteries concerning smallpox is how and why variolation developed. An accidental inoculation of the virus through the skin, through an open cut or sore, would not have been noticed in smallpox-endemic areas, so it must have been done consciously and deliberately. A clinical trial of sorts would have been required to detect the difference in mortality rates for those inoculated compared to those who acquired smallpox by natural spread. In any case, variolation was practiced for centuries, right up into the 1960s and the days of the smallpox eradication program. In fact, smallpox eradication workers had to be alert to the possibility of variolation because it was one way of initiating smallpox outbreaks.

Variolation was apparently practiced in Africa well before colonial rule. A Hausa woman, recalling her childhood in the 1890s, described a method of passing the disease "from arm to arm." She said, "They used to scratch your arm until the blood came, then they got the fluid from someone who had the smallpox and rubbed it in. It all swelled up and you covered it until you healed. Some children used to die; your way of doing it is better."[8]

During the colonial era, variolation did make its way to Europe and North America. The colorful American clergyman Cotton Mather, possessed of a scientific mind, observed that the black population of Boston had a lower attack rate for smallpox than did the whites. He discovered that slaves had brought the practice of variolation from Africa and were using it to protect themselves. In his enthusiasm, he wrote a tract promoting the practice. Many, however, believed that variolation actually spread the disease (which it could) and that, moreover, it was against God's will. The practice never took firm root in the New World. In Britain, meanwhile, Lady Montague, wife of the British ambassador to Turkey, reported in 1717 on the Turkish use of variolation; her account interested the royal family enough that they decided to try it—first on criminals and only then on their own children. It became accepted in Britain and was practiced widely.

In West Africa, variolation was performed by practitioners called *fetisheurs*. In 1969, while visiting Benin (then called Dahomey) in connection with the eradication program, I spent a day with one practitioner. He looked like a typical village person but was better dressed. He exuded the confidence of a person who knows more than those around him, though without the arrogance often seen in city dwellers who returned to their villages for a visit. He enjoyed talking, and through an interpreter, answered my most probing questions with candor and clarity. Indeed, he reminded me of an attending physician teaching a medical student.

The *fetisheur*, it became clear, knew exactly what he was doing. When a person had smallpox, the family would consult him. He would instruct the patient on what he or she needed to do to recover. The *fetisheur* knew that the mortality rate for smallpox in his area was between 20 and 25 percent; he also knew that most of his patients would therefore recover, regardless of treatment. The *fetisheur* was rewarded by the family either way. If the patient died, he simply informed the family that the patient had not followed his very specific instructions.

Fetisheurs, this practitioner explained, used visits to patients as opportunities to collect scabs, which they kept in bottles in a dark place, having discovered that sunlight and heat render the virus impotent. If no smallpox had occurred for some time and a *fetisheur* needed business, he could seed an outbreak by what amounted to covert variolation. He would grind scabs into a paste, coat thorn branches with the paste, and place these in doorways where they would scratch unsuspecting passersby. Even a single "take" could start a new outbreak.

In due course, the practitioner introduced me to his two students, who were serving two-year "residencies" to learn the trade. Their knowledge of smallpox and its transmission was impressive. In their efforts to understand and communicate about the cause of the disease, however, the *fetisheurs* did not use what we in the West would call a scientific approach. Rather, they told patients that they had contracted the disease because they were being punished for some previous offense. When I asked why babies, too young to have committed misdeeds, sometimes contracted the disease, the three men responded almost in unison: the baby was being punished for something the parents had done.

The disappearance of smallpox from West Africa was bad for business, and the *fetisheurs* did not give up their smallpox enterprise without a fight. Multiple *fetisheurs* visited the last smallpox patient in Benin in order to harvest scabs, but they were unable to propagate the virus, and smallpox disappeared despite their best efforts. Adapting to market changes, some began to consult on cases of chickenpox, with a high success rate for recovery.

FOUR

Fire Line around a Virus

As planned, my family and I traveled to Atlanta at the beginning of July 1966. I participated in the CDC training course and in October returned to Nigeria. Paula, with four-year-old David and our newborn, Michael, followed a few weeks later. This time we settled in Enugu, Eastern Nigeria's capital. We rented a second-floor flat that had both running water and electricity, which after Okpoma and Yahe seemed like luxuries. I would work with the smallpox program during the week and commute back to Yahe some weekends to work at the clinic.

The shift from village to town offered a new perspective on the culture of Africa. Villages operate by unwritten rules understood by all, and the people are generally friendly and helpful. While the rhythm of life is hard, it is also soothing. The village is also safe. I could be gone overnight and not have to worry about my family. Indeed, the villagers provided a night watchman for our house, demonstrating that they would look out for us. Urban living offers amenities—it was a heady experience to buy food in a store or go to a British-style club for a swim after work—yet it is also faster, more crowded, and less socially cohesive. Those who move to the cities can lose touch with the rules of village life and even lose their way entirely. Later during our stay, a burglar entered through our second-floor window and took cameras and valuables, including money from the pocket of trousers hanging next to our occupied bed.

In a poor urban setting like Enugu, everyone is scrambling daily for some small advantage. Several weeks into our stay in Enugu, Lawrence Atutu Ochelebe, who had moved with us from Yahe and was both clever and fiercely loyal, told me that he thought a neighbor might have tapped into our electrical line. While this might be seen as stealing, in very poor societies successfully tapping into an electrical line can also be admired as a small victory. Nonetheless, it was unacceptable. Lawrence and I decided to test his hypothesis by having him turn off our main electrical input line after sunset while I watched the neighbors' lights. I was surprised to watch multiple flats go dark!

Similarly, one Saturday night as Paula and I returned to our flat after attending a movie, I noticed one of the smallpox trucks—unmistakable white Dodge crew cabs with large backseats and pickup beds—stopped at an intersection and loaded high with household effects. I knew that all three of our vehicles should have been in the Ministry of Health garage. The driver was making extra money by using it as a moving van. On Monday morning, at the end of the weekly staff meeting, I mentioned that I would like the driver who had been out with one of the trucks at 10 P.M. on Saturday night to stay behind. All three drivers stayed behind! We reviewed the rules, but people in need are under such pressure to find creative ways to get by that it is very difficult to totally stop such activities.

In late November of 1966, the CDC assignees—David Thompson, accompanied by his wife, Joan, and Paul Lichfield, with his wife, Mary— joined Paula and me in Enugu. David, Paul, and I were assigned to work with the regional Ministry of Health to eradicate smallpox from the Eastern Region, an area of 12 million people. We immediately began making plans to train teams and fan them out across the region to vaccinate the entire population area by area.

We were helped by two aspects of the culture. First, the people in the region, and in West Africa generally, placed high value on injections. In recent years AIDS has changed that attitude, but in the 1960s injections were regarded with such favor that there was a large underground movement of illicit injection programs. At the medical center at Yahe, I discovered while treating a large abscess in a patient's buttock that he had recently received an injection from the medical center's carpenter, who was taking supplies from our pharmacy and running a thriving injection practice at night. The popularity of injections may have originated with the first village-to-village programs in the late 1940s, which sought out people with yaws and treated them with penicillin injections. The effect of the penicillin was dramatic; the unsightly chronic sores healed quickly. The injection, rather than the penicillin, was credited as powerful.

Second, community leaders—schoolteachers, local health workers, and political or religious leaders—provided valuable assistance in setting up vaccination sites and educating the public. People feared smallpox and for the most part understood that we were offering vaccinations to prevent it. I have no doubt, though, that many were vaccinated not because our information convinced them but because they trusted their leaders, who supported the vaccination effort.

As an example, sometime in 1967 after the vaccination program was well under way, I stopped in a village to set up a time for vaccinations. Through an interpreter I told the chief I could make sure his village was protected against smallpox if he could persuade them to be vaccinated. He agreed, and I asked when he would like to do it. He surprised me by saying, "Let's do it right now." "But," I protested, "people are out working in the fields at the moment. I would be happy to return late in the day." He insisted he could get them to return for something this important, and he spoke to an assistant, who began beating a talking drum.

People began streaming into this large village, and with a jet injector I vaccinated several thousand in a few hours. Afterward, I sat down with the chief and remarked on his ability to get the entire village to respond so quickly. I asked him about the talking drum. Through it, had he communicated a set signal to return to the village, or had he sent a more specific message? He assured me it was a specific message. I asked him what he had said, and he replied, "I told them to come to the market if they wanted to see the tallest man in the world." At six feet seven inches, I don't actually qualify, but it was enough to get the desired result.

Intrigued by the talking drums, I later had the opportunity to test their precision. I was sitting with a drummer in a village, and two men, one wearing a green shirt and the other wearing a blue shirt, were standing at a distance too far away to hear us talking. I asked the drummer to direct the man wearing the blue shirt to ask the man wearing the green shirt if he could borrow the pen clipped to his shirt pocket. The drummer began drumming, and the instructions were carried out exactly.

THE WHO SMALLPOX ERADICATION PROGRAM

The eradication effort in Eastern Nigeria was one small part of a program the CDC had agreed to administer for the WHO. D. A. Henderson, who had earned a stellar reputation at the CDC for his work in developing disease surveillance programs, had been influential in the development of WHO's smallpox eradication program. Once the program was approved, Henderson was detailed from CDC to the WHO headquarters in Geneva to supervise the global effort. Henderson's assignment turned out to be crucial for smallpox eradication. Not only was he skillful in negotiating global agreements and alliances, but his origins at CDC meant a steady influx of CDC people, as well as CDC investment, in the global program over the next decade.

The CDC was charged with interrupting smallpox transmission in twenty designated countries of West and Central Africa within five years, with funding provided by the U.S. Agency for International Development (USAID). This area of Africa, geographically larger than the United States, was considered at the time to be the toughest smallpox region in the world. It had the highest smallpox rates (number of cases per thousand population) in the world, according to WHO figures, as well as the poorest health infrastructure, transportation, and communication facilities. Since measles was the single most lethal agent in Africa in the 1960s, the program targeted measles as well. Measles vaccines had entered the armamentarium of public health in the developed countries, and USAID now offered the vaccine to West and Central Africa. Children between six months and six years of age were to receive measles vaccine, while the entire population would receive smallpox vaccine.

Don Millar, who had worked with Henderson to lay the groundwork for the global smallpox program, was put in charge of the Africa program.[1] Don brought considerable enthusiasm to whatever task he took on. In his new role as director of the Africa program, Don showed great leadership abilities as he recruited, trained, and dispatched some forty medical and operations officers to West Africa. He also brought a strong respect for evidence to the job. He constantly reviewed what was working and why, reporting his observations weekly in a newsletter called "Friday Afternoon Reflections," and he was always ready to implement successful new tactics in place of what wasn't working.

Since the days of Jefferson and Jenner, people had thought that smallpox should be eradicable. By the mid-1960s, enough countries had become free of smallpox that it was clear that the vaccine, if applied correctly, could bring about eradication. However, eradication had so far been accomplished only in wealthy countries and in countries with a low level of smallpox or with smallpox workers who were obsessive in pursuing the program. What remained unknown was whether the same goal could be accomplished in poor countries that had high smallpox rates combined with meager health resources and inadequate infrastructures and communications systems.

Some people assumed that it could be done, that it was just a matter of addressing the inherent problems of resource-poor nations. Others maintained that smallpox could never be eradicated, and they offered as proof the fact that similar efforts to eradicate malaria as well as yellow fever had failed. Those who believed eradication was possible would point out the difference: unlike malaria and yellow fever, smallpox is entirely dependent on human organisms in its life cycle. The doubters would respond that no disease had ever before been eradicated, and thus it was surely an impossible goal.

It was in this climate of hope, doubt, and debate that the WHA executive board finally approved a global smallpox eradication project in

February 1966. This decision did not come easily. Back in 1958, the Soviet Union had proposed before the WHA a resolution calling for a global effort to eradicate smallpox. The resolution had passed, but little in the way of substantial efforts had followed. At its May 1965 meeting, the WHA again debated the issue. Many countries, including the USSR and the United States, supported the idea, but there was disagreement over how to budget for the program, and once again the delegates passed a resolution with no plan for action. The following year, in 1966, the WHA finally ratified a funded program for global smallpox eradication, to be completed within ten years, and asked WHO to assume the principal role in organizing and coordinating the effort.[2]

There were several reasons why the WHO program had a good chance of succeeding. First, key technological advances made it possible to standardize the quality and stability of the smallpox vaccine worldwide. Up to this time, the production of the vaccine had remained almost a cottage industry in many countries. This meant that while the vaccinia virus—somewhat modified over the years from Jenner's original cowpox virus—was a great vaccine, it wasn't consistently great. The potency varied widely. The production process was crude, involving shaving calves, scarifying the exposed skin (scratching or lacerating the skin to make it raw), and painting this raw surface with a substance containing vaccinia virus. The virus would grow on the scarified tissue and then be harvested by raking off the pustular material. The resulting matter was cleaned of extraneous bits of hair and flesh to provide high concentrations of vaccinia virus. It looked as unappetizing as it sounds.

Much of the resulting vaccine was kept in a liquid form that required refrigeration to remain viable—yet high temperatures were the norm in most smallpox-endemic areas. It was possible to launch effective programs with liquid vaccine, as many areas had shown over 160 years, but it was very difficult. Early in the twentieth century a method was developed for freeze-drying vaccines, permitting them to be stored at room temperature for extended periods. However, there remained the problem of how to convert all the vaccinia manufacturers around the world to this new technology.

Early in the eradication program, WHO, under the leadership of D. A.

Henderson, assembled a panel of experts who came up with a global standard for the vaccine and created a detailed manual for its production as well as how to convert to freeze-drying the vaccine. Consultants were sent out to help countries convert to the new system. Reference centers for testing vaccines were established in Canada and the Netherlands. To fill the gap while all areas of the world were catching up, two dozen countries already producing vaccine of satisfactory quality donated vaccine where it was needed. By 1969, all vaccine used in the smallpox-endemic countries met WHO standards, and by 1973 more than 80 percent of the vaccine in use was being produced by the developing countries themselves.

A simplified and improved vaccination technique, in the form of the jet injector, also increased the odds of success for the global eradication effort. Up to the mid-twentieth century, most areas of the world were still using the multiple pressure vaccination technique, in which a vaccinator repeatedly pressed a needle, at an angle, through a drop of vaccine placed on the vaccinee's skin. The needle nicked the skin on the upstroke, created a small injured area where the vaccine could begin multiplying. The procedure is simple but difficult to teach, which meant that take rates varied according to the vaccinator's skill and even for the same vaccinator under different conditions. The method also required cleaning the skin before vaccination, which meant that vaccinators were encumbered with bottles of alcohol, acetone, or soap and cotton swabs.

Another method still used in some countries, including India, was the rotary lancet. This brutal instrument consisted of a quarter-inch-diameter wheel with tines attached to a long axle. The wheel was placed on the vaccinee's skin and the axle was rotated by the vaccinator's fingers, causing cuts as the tines rotated through a drop of vaccine, giving the vaccine access to underlying tissue. The result, once the vaccine took and the lesion healed, was a large vaccination scar. Many vaccinators would do two or three vaccinations on the vaccinee's forearm or upper arm to increase the chances that one would take. In fact, if the vaccine was not potent, none of the attempts would provide a take; if it was potent, the person was likely to end up with more than one hot, angry vaccination lesion developing at the same time.

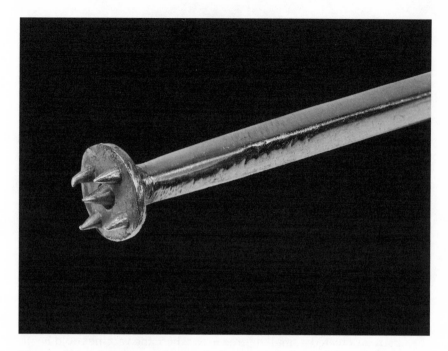

Figure 3. Rotary lancet, a vaccination device used in India until the early 1970s. CDC/Bruce Weniger; James Gathany

In 1960, Aaron Ismach, working with the U.S. Army, had developed a foot-operated jet injector, called the Ped-O-Jet, that was an efficient work of art. It consisted of a hydraulic foot pedal that, with a single step, depressed a piston releasing just enough pressure for one vaccination. The vaccinator placed the pistol-like portion of the jet injector against the vaccinee's skin and pulled the trigger, releasing a plunger that delivered the vaccine intradermally, between the layers of the skin. No needle was involved. A 50 cc bottle attached to the injector could provide five hundred doses of 0.1 cc smallpox vaccine.

The jet injector's tidy and reliable delivery of a packet of virus allowed for uniform take rates (approaching 100 percent) even with different vaccinators. The technique was simple and quickly learned, and because there was so little wastage, the Ped-O-Jet was economical. The 1964

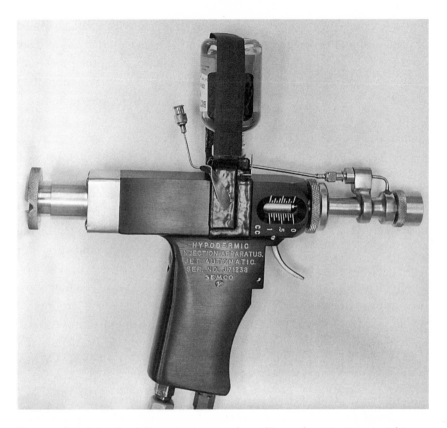

Figure 4. Ped-O-Jet, the delivery instrument for millions of vaccinations in Africa in the 1960s. CDC/Susan Lindsley

Tonga study I had participated in had determined an effective dilution rate for the vaccine, which meant additional savings.

The Ped-O-Jet, introduced into the West Africa program in late 1966, made it possible to vaccinate one thousand people in an hour. On one occasion, while vaccinating in a large prison where the prisoners moved past the injector in a highly disciplined way, we were able to deliver six hundred vaccinations in less than thirty minutes. During one very long day in Enugu, I did 11,600 vaccinations.

The Ped-O-Jet's speed offered little advantage if vaccinators moved house to house. Instead, arrangements were made with a village ahead of time, and on the designated day, the vaccinators would arrive and set up the site. People often milled around the site watching the procedure before committing to participate. Even after their own vaccination, they would stay around to watch others go through the line, pressing in to the point where we could no longer move people past the injector. Crowd control was essential. If the site was under a tree, we delineated the route people should take with ropes wrapped around three-foot metal stakes. If it was in a church or school, the vaccinator would be positioned immediately inside the doorway so only one person at a time could pass by.

In addition to these technological advances, the new world order that had emerged after World War II, particularly the development of the United Nations and WHO, made it practical to consider and carry out global objectives. The idea of a global perspective was not new. The Greek historian Polybius understood two thousand years ago that nothing happens in isolation. He said the world must be seen as an organic whole, and he provided examples of events in Africa impacting Athens. By the mid-twentieth century, a global view could truly include the entire world. The UN and WHO made it possible, for the first time in history, to select a global health objective, organize to reach that objective, and apply the greatest resources to the largest problems.

A global perspective is essential to dealing with infectious diseases, since diseases have no regard for national boundaries. And, it turns out, what's good for the global community is good for the individual country. For the United States, which had been smallpox-free since 1949, the investment in global smallpox eradication amounted to just one-quarter of the annual expense of vaccinating U.S. children and maintaining a program to check the vaccination status of people coming into the country.

A less tangible yet no less important ingredient in smallpox eradication was simply the belief that it could be done. In fact, in retrospect, the belief that it could be done seems like the most important factor in the global eradication effort. The technology and the infrastructure were necessary, but the planning and hard work required to use them to full effect rested on the faith that eradication was possible. We all know the adage that some things have to be seen to be believed. In fact, the opposite is often true: some things have to be believed to be seen.

The fact of smallpox was so ingrained in human experience that we had our work cut out for us to convince people that eradication was not a wishful fantasy. The shift from doubt to belief was not unlike a religious conversion; it involved not just facts, but emotion, too. A person suddenly transformed by the vision of what was possible could not be stopped. One dramatic example was Dr. George Glokpur, head of the smallpox eradication program for Togo. In 1967, he attended a three-week course on smallpox eradication held at the CDC in Atlanta. After the first week, he decided to go home. By then, he was convinced he could do it and did not want to wait an additional two weeks before getting started.

As more geographic areas became free of smallpox, it became easier to transmit this belief. Like a communicable disease, the belief in smallpox eradication was infectious, with an incubation period, various degrees of susceptibility, and an increasing rate of spread that finally infected many who came in its path. Once this condition was shared by a critical mass of people, no barrier was insurmountable.

Even though we were setting out to do something never accomplished before, we believed, from the beginning, that eradication of this disease was possible. What we did not know was that we yet lacked a key ingredient: a more effective primary strategy. This final element was fortuitously discovered at the very outset of the program.

CHANGING THE PRIMARY STRATEGY

As the CDC smallpox eradication teams established programs in West and Central Africa in late 1966 and into 1967, they followed the same plan that vaccinators had followed for seventeen decades: to vaccinate as many people as possible. This method provided direct protection for the person vaccinated and aimed to accomplish "herd immunity"—indirect protection for unvaccinated persons who would have acquired smallpox if the vaccinated person had become sick. There is no question that mass vaccination could work, as was demonstrated early on in Ceylon (now

Sri Lanka) and later in Bolivia, China, and in many countries of the industrialized world.

The problem with mass vaccination is that an exceedingly obsessive program is required to make inroads into the last 20 percent of any population. The segments of the population most difficult to reach with vaccine—the drifters, the marginalized populations, beggars, itinerant workers—are often the ones most at risk of both getting and spreading the disease. Therefore, surveillance and containment of outbreaks was seen as the next step after mass vaccination. Add to this the high population densities in urban areas and it becomes clear that herd immunity is easy in theory but not fully effective in practice. Even with a good program, a critical mass of unprotected persons can accumulate, and the vulnerability of such unvaccinated pockets often leads to an explosive outbreak when the smallpox virus is reintroduced. This problem is well recognized in public health. Yet at the time it was the best plan anyone had. My CDC colleagues and I working in Eastern Nigeria embraced this strategy, and during the final months of 1966 began making plans to pursue it with determination.

Serendipity provided a chance for us to rethink the eradication strategy before the year ended. On December 4, 1966, Hector Ottemüller, a longtime missionary in the Ogoja area, contacted me by radio. There was an outbreak of smallpox in the village of Ovirpua, in the Alifokpa area of Ogoja province, some ninety miles northeast of Enugu, and Hector was asking if the smallpox unit could help. Ottemüller was a minister by training, with a patriarchal bearing enhanced by striking white hair and a white beard. His consuming interest lay in improving the lives of the people in his rural area. He was involved in agriculture and water supply schemes, although the people also called upon him for health advice. Thus it was not surprising that he was the first to receive the report of a rash disease feared by all in his area.

The village of Ovirpua was some miles from a road, but Dave Thompson and I managed to get hold of two Solex motorbikes, which were ideal for this work. Made in France, they are essentially sturdy bicycles with a small motor that engages directly on the rubber of the front tire, and they are lightweight enough to be carried under one arm

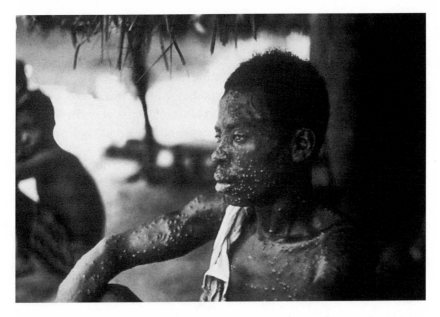

Figure 5. First smallpox patient seen in Ogoja, Nigeria, outbreak, December 4, 1966

across logs spanning creeks. We arrived at Ovirpua in mid-afternoon. The first person I examined was a young man in his twenties, and there was no question about the diagnosis. We examined and questioned four other people who had the disease. We vaccinated the patients' family members and other villagers in immediate contact with them.

That night, Thompson and I and several missionaries assembled around kerosene lamps in the house of a missionary who lived in the area. We talked through the problem while educating the missionaries about the sobering situation we were facing. We knew this was smallpox but we did not know its extent. How many villages were involved? How many people were sick and how many were in the incubation period? Had it just been introduced to the area, or had it been smoldering for some time?

The standard response was to vaccinate everyone within a certain radius while attempting to determine the extent of the outbreak. However, we did not have enough vaccine to do this. The program was so new that supplies had not yet arrived in quantity, and there was no likelihood of quickly receiving more. How could we most efficiently use the limited amount of vaccine we had on hand?

It was tempting to consider diluting the vaccine so we could vaccinate more people. However, history showed that this was a risk that should not be taken. In 1962, Dr. Robert Hingson, founder of the Brother's Brother Foundation, committed to vaccinate Liberia's population of about 1.3 million people against smallpox. A massive campaign was undertaken, but the program organizers found that they had underestimated their vaccine needs, so they diluted the vaccine fifteen-fold. A subsequent assessment by WHO indicated that only 60 to 70 percent of the population had successful primary vaccinations, and 325 cases of smallpox were reported in Liberia the same year, after the campaign ended.[3] Some people who had been vaccinated subsequently got smallpox, probably because of the vaccine dilution. If we now did the same thing, we could be leaving unprotected an unknown number of people who were directly in the viral path.

Forced to look for another solution, we raised the question: if we were smallpox viruses bent on immortality, what would we do to extend our family tree? The answer of course was to find the nearest susceptible person in which to continue reproduction. Our task, then, was not to vaccinate everyone within a certain range but rather to identify and protect the nearest susceptible people before the virus could reach them.

What we knew about the virus's behavior also figured into our strategy. The smallpox virus poses little risk to people other than its host during the incubation period. It is only when the characteristic sores form on the skin and mucous membranes that the virus can escape the host and seek new victims. Spread is also easiest during the early days of rash, when the number of virus particles on the body's surfaces is large and people may not yet recognize the disease. The potential for spread decreases as people become wary, and as the host's immune mechanisms respond and the number of viruses on the patient's exterior declines. Spread is most likely within the first week of clinical symptoms and is probably rare after three weeks.

We discussed the risks of spread. The highest spread potential was obviously in the home, but early in the illness the patients might also have been in contact with visiting relatives or might have attended one of the region's markets. We could use the missionaries' knowledge of market patterns and family patterns to make predictions about high-risk areas for spread, but first we needed to know where the virus was at that moment.

Acquiring this type of intelligence would be difficult even in a country like the United States. It seemed absolutely impossible in rural Africa. However, the missionary community's own support system offered an answer. There were no telephones, so every night at 7 P.M., the missionaries turned on their shortwave radios and checked in to make sure that no one was in need of assistance.

We weren't that hopeful, but it was worth a try. That night we got on the radio with missionaries up to some thirty or more miles distant, explained the situation, and, with maps in front of us, divided up the area. We asked each missionary to send runners to every village in his assigned area to ask if anyone had seen cases of smallpox.

The following night Thompson and the local missionaries and I again got on the radio, and to our joy and amazement were given the precise information we needed. Only four villages had smallpox cases at that moment. The rest were free of the disease.

Our plan was straightforward. First, we vaccinated the currently infected villages, where some people were probably already infected even if they had not yet developed symptoms. For those recently exposed, vaccination would greatly reduce the disease's impact, if not prevent it. Those exposed even two weeks earlier would still get smallpox, but they would be surrounded by vaccinated people, making further transmission of the virus very difficult. If we were fortunate, it might even stop transmission totally.

Second, based on the missionaries' knowledge of where the patients and their families usually traveled, we made some informed guesses regarding other places where the virus was most likely incubating. We identified three, all within a fifteen-mile radius, and decided to use the remaining vaccine there. We could not know as we vaccinated these three additional areas that smallpox was already incubating in two of them. By

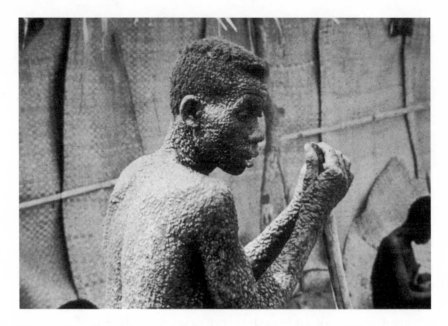

Figure 6. Patient outside the infectious disease hut near Abakaliki, Nigeria, 1967

the time clinical cases were detected in these two places, the remaining population was already protected—and smallpox was stopped in its tracks. The outcome was the complete cessation of this outbreak.

"Life accumulates" was a favorite saying of Jim Laney, former president of Emory University. In many ways the strategy that stopped the virus was a logical extension of the firefighting principle I was taught back in the summers of 1956 and 1957. By removing the fuel one step ahead of the virus, we had built a fire line around it.

A BETTER WAY

Dave Thompson, Paul Lichfield, and I had no way of knowing that this new approach was going to work as well as it did, so during the subsequent weeks as the scenario in Ogoja province unfolded, we acquired more vaccine and, with the help of the missionaries, expanded vaccination coverage in the area. However, once the transmission ceased, we realized that these additional vaccinations, while building herd immunity against a future outbreak, did nothing to stop the current outbreak. If smallpox never returned to this area (and it never did), then every additional vaccination was essentially wasted effort—a theft of time and vaccine. Even on this small scale, we were seeing the inefficiency of mass vaccination.

Despite this success, we did not immediately abandon the mass vaccination approach. Indeed, we went ahead and implemented it because that is what we had been sent to do. After Christmas, we began training teams of health workers from the Eastern Nigeria Ministry of Health. We used stopwatches to see how fast they could set up an immunization site, drive in stakes, attach ropes for crowd control, clean the jet injectors, set up one injector for smallpox vaccine and another for measles vaccine, and when all was in order, give the first immunization. The teams became proficient and even competitive in demonstrating their skills.

Once the teams were trained, we ran a vaccination pilot project in Abakaliki, a city located east of Enugu. The project was nearly perfection in execution, community involvement was high, and our evaluations showed that we had vaccinated over 94 percent of the population, an incredible coverage rate at any time but especially impressive as a first effort.

We had barely finished congratulating ourselves when a smallpox outbreak was reported in Abakaliki. We were sure there must be some mistake, but investigation confirmed that it was definitely smallpox. We figured that the outbreak was in a small geographic pocket of people that had somehow been missed. But as the number of cases mounted, we were surprised to find them distributed throughout the city. All of the infected people turned out to be members of a religious group, the Faith Tabernacle Church, that had refused vaccinations based on religious convictions. They comprised a missed pocket but not a geographic pocket.

This experience altered our thinking. Clearly, mass vaccination could protect the vast majority of a population without guaranteeing that smallpox transmission would cease. This reinforced the lesson of the Ogoja outbreak—that there might be a better way.

FIVE Extinguishing Smallpox in a Time of War

In the first weeks of 1967, Dave Thompson, Paul Lichfield, and I made a choice we could not have predicted. As we designed the eradication project for Nigeria's Eastern Region, we also researched smallpox reports from past years. We recorded the previous outbreaks by date and place on maps of the region, and as we did, a macro pattern appeared. At the beginning of most high-transmission seasons, smallpox outbreaks were generally more prevalent in the northern part of Eastern Nigeria, suggesting that they migrated in from the Northern Region and gradually moved southward. We wondered initially if we could impede the progression, and thus stop smallpox, by building a fire line of mass vaccinations across the northern part of the region. The results in Abakaliki, however, were compelling and gave us pause, especially as they followed so soon after the dramatic results in Ogoja. We decided that the surveillance/containment approach ought to be tested in a larger area.

With this thought in mind, we talked with Dr. A. Anezanwu, director of the smallpox program for the Eastern Region and our supervisor at the Ministry of Health in Enugu, about putting most of our resources into surveillance and containment, focusing on the northern portion of the region first, with plans to continue south. We would go ahead with some mass vaccination activities because the measles program required that approach. But we could channel much of our effort into finding and containing outbreaks as the mass vaccination approach proceeded. Changing strategies involved risk. If the new strategy failed, the entire Nigerian eradication program could possibly be delayed or even jeopardized. As we discussed the pros and cons, Dr. Anezanwu warmed to the idea of trying something new and radical. He was a member of the Ibo tribe, as were the majority of people in the Eastern Region, and the Ibos have a reputation for entrepreneurship and taking risks. He agreed to try surveillance/containment, though probably not because we were so persuasive. Rather, Eastern Nigeria in early 1967 was the right place and time for decisions that were at odds with federal thinking. It was yet another expression of the rebellion brewing at that time.

TESTING A RADICAL APPROACH
IN A REBELLIOUS LAND

What no one knew was that we had only six months to test the new approach. War was looming between the Eastern Region and the rest of Nigeria. When we consulted political officers about how soon the fighting would start, they were somewhat reassuring: both sides needed time to secure weapons, train soldiers, and actually begin military actions; meanwhile, there were hopes for a settlement that would forestall war.

The political situation affected the smallpox effort directly. For one thing, it increased the risks involved in travel. The fear of war meant heightened security and numerous local roadblocks. On some trips, our car was stopped and searched every few miles. The roadblocks were often maintained by citizen soldiers or two or three teenagers who mixed guns, alcohol, and bravado. They had to be taken seriously at all times. Sometimes travel was facilitated by showing an official letter that stated our purpose and asked all security personnel to speed our travel for the sake of stopping smallpox. This might not work if the guards lacked sufficient literacy, but the reverse was also true: someone wanting to fake literacy would feign reading an official-looking letter and give orders to allow us to proceed. We soon learned to construct our own letters, putting enough stamps on them so they conveyed importance.

One missionary was questioned at a roadblock about the labeling machine in the trunk of her car. She explained its use and then demonstrated it by asking one guard for his name, which she spelled out on a label. She presented the label to the very happy young man, and of course the other two guards requested the same and she obliged. Several miles beyond the roadblock she became aware of an unusual rattling noise, so she stopped the car and opened the trunk. Three AK-47s were piled in the trunk, left by the guards as they walked off admiring their name tags. When she appeared again at the roadblock, the young men were visibly relieved; with their weapons returned, their supervisor wouldn't discover that they had been disarmed.

On one occasion when I was traveling, the driver discovered just as we approached a roadblock that the brakes were not working, nor was the emergency brake. No one would even consider running a roadblock, so the driver jerked the steering wheel to the right, our van hit the ditch hard, proceeded up the other side, knocked down a small tree, and came to rest against a mud hut. A crowd began to gather around us, and soon the area chief arrived. Once he had sized up the predicament, he spoke through an interpreter, telling a story in the powerful oratorical style prized in Africa. The story went on for some time, but the bottom line was that our truck had hit a sacred juju tree. This had offended the juju gods and would require the sacrifice of a chicken, which cost 10 shillings, and he expected me to pay. My initial emotion was relief. Ten shillings was a small price to pay, and we could be on our way.

However, something perverse invaded my thinking, and before I had thought it through, I began to respond. I had every intention of paying the 10 shillings. I also knew from experience that the chief was very likely taking advantage of the situation—the tree was probably not a juju tree, but as a visitor I had no option but to pay. I explained that in my culture, the van had some of the characteristics of a juju god, and the truck was offended that the tree was in its way. I would now have to sacrifice a goat, which cost 20 shillings. I pulled 10 shillings from my pocket and asked who would receive my 10 shillings and who would give me the 20 shillings. The silence was so heavy that I immediately knew I had made a big mistake. But then one man broke the silence with a laugh. It was contagious and soon everyone was laughing. No money changed hands, everyone joked about who was the biggest storyteller, and we were off in low gear to find a place to fix our broken brake line.

ACQUIRING CRUCIAL SUPPLIES

The political tensions at times forced us to take risks just to accomplish our job. The Nigerian federal health authorities now questioned everything being done in the Eastern Region, including the rapid start of its smallpox program. This was evident at a meeting called in Lagos in early 1967 to discuss health education for Nigeria's smallpox eradication program. The meeting was disintegrating into a full-blown attack on the posters, methods, and plans in the Eastern Region, when a young professor from the University of Ibaden, Dr. Adetokunbo Lucas, commented that a prime objective of health education is to get the attention of people in order to transmit a message, and that the Eastern Nigeria materials had just attracted more attention than materials from any other region. That simple observation by a person of distinction from a non–Eastern Nigeria tribe brought the meeting back to its purpose. Lucas would go on to have a distinguished career, with posts at WHO, the Carnegie Corporation, and Harvard University.

The federal authorities nevertheless decided it was time to rein in Eastern Nigeria's smallpox effort. Explaining that the country must work in a unified way, the federal government cut off smallpox supplies to the Eastern Region—until the other regions had caught up. We were now faced with the serious matter of inadequate supplies—even for a new strategy that was based on a shortage of supplies. Such difficulties were not just bothersome; they threatened the very existence of the program. Moreover, lives were at risk if we had no means to stop existing outbreaks.

In March 1967, as supplies were running short, I drove to Lagos one day with another CDC team member and a plan. We needed some jet injector parts. Requesting these was not likely to be a problem since they were maintenance items, not supplies. In the meantime, we could learn how the warehouse system worked and get to know the warehouse security people. As it turned out, during our visit, one of us kept the security person engaged in trying to find specific items while the other person was free to quietly and furtively acquire essential supplies. We loaded the white Dodge pickup with vaccine, diluent, cold boxes, cold packs, jet injector parts, and anything else we thought we would need to continue the campaign. We now had a truck full of the items that the Nigerian federal government had denied us—and we were scared.

A more direct approach might have been to bribe a security person. But including one additional person in the plan might have caused it to unravel, and there would be no second chance. Indeed, we decided not to even inform the CDC supervisor in Lagos, in case his work would be compromised if it ever came to light that he was aware of our activity. While I always suspected that he was aware of and understood the importance of our actions, the approach of simply taking what we needed is still sufficiently distasteful that in the forty years since then I have never discussed the event with him.

By midmorning my colleague and I were on our way back to Enugu, and we were more than nervous. We didn't even stop for food, as we imagined that shortages had been discovered by now and a posse had been formed to bring us to justice. Every vehicle approaching from behind was a source of fear.

In truth, no one even noticed. Months later, our supervisor mentioned some difficulty the federal smallpox program was having with its inventory. If this was an attempt to get us to open up, it did not work. I continued to believe that he supported our effort by keeping quiet.

We made it to the Onitsha Bridge, still several hours from Enugu, just as it was getting dark. The Onitsha was the only bridge across the Niger River for the entire western border of the Eastern Region. If we couldn't cross there, we would have to drive more than one hundred miles north to take a ferry across the river.

We found the bridge blocked with bulldozers and trucks. The people of the Eastern Region were worried about a federal invasion from the west. We drove up to the bridge's entrance and asked the guards if we could speak with the commanding officer. They referred us to their superior, and up the chain of command we went, finally getting to a person with the authority required. We explained our situation and that we needed to get back to Enugu in time to refrigerate the vaccines. The commander asked his men to move the vehicles enough so we could pass, and we were able to wind our way through the roadblock and continue on to Enugu, arriving after midnight.

Hindsight brings clarity. In retrospect, obtaining those supplies from the warehouse in Lagos looms as one of the essential actions in a decade of events leading to smallpox eradication worldwide. In the extended chain of events from success in surveillance/containment in Ogoja province to the interruption of smallpox transmission with the help of this strategy in Africa, India, and elsewhere, perhaps no link in the chain was as precarious as proving that surveillance/containment could work as the primary strategy for an entire region. This happened in Eastern Nigeria, thanks to adequate supplies.

WAR LOOMS

Through the first half of 1967, the smallpox team in Eastern Nigeria identified every outbreak of smallpox in the region and contained each one in turn. We were now confirming, through what amounted to additional field-testing, that the theory of vaccinating only those who were at immediate risk of exposure was sound. However, the strategy was new, and we were still unsure about how large an area of vaccination was required to contain an outbreak, so we tended to err on the side of excess. When smallpox cases were admitted to the Enugu hospital, we opted for a rapid mass vaccination program for the entire city. We believed that even in this situation the surveillance/containment approach, with the identification and vaccination of all contacts, would have been enough to stop transmission. But lack of experience made us cautious.

We learned of the hospital cases on a Saturday and immediately made plans to have vaccination teams in place to begin the urban campaign in less than forty-eight hours. I traveled through the city that afternoon, looking for vacant lots where we could set up vaccination posts and marking them on a large-scale map of the city. I became totally engrossed in the process of balancing the location of vacant lots with easy access for people and minimal disruption of the usual activities while envisioning how the teams would move, how long they would remain at each vaccination site, and the number of people required per team. I hadn't thought about the fact that what I was doing might appear suspicious. Suddenly I was surrounded by armed police and placed under arrest. I learned that day that egress is more difficult than access when it comes to jails. Six hours later, the police finally allowed me to contact the Ministry of Health, and my Nigerian counterpart came to the jail to secure my release.

Throughout the early months of 1967, as we were successfully containing outbreaks, belligerent talk filled the newspapers. The Eastern Region threatened to leave Nigeria to form a new country, and the federal government promised military action if such an attempt was made. Tensions increased following the killing of Ibos in Northern Nigeria, and refugees began to flow into the Eastern Region. Amid the charges and countercharges, many groups tried to start peace talks even as both sides desperately tried to improve their military capability. Paula and I decided that in the event of violence in Enugu, we and our two children would stay in our upstairs flat. We had enough canned food on hand to feed us for several weeks. We agreed that at the first sign of trouble, we would fill our bathtub with water for drinking and cooking in case municipal water supplies were interrupted.

One Saturday in March, it was announced repeatedly on the radio that military maneuvers would be conducted at midnight and the streets should be vacated. The announcements were not in English, and in any event we were not listening to the radio, so we were unaware of the exercise. At midnight, shortly after I had fallen asleep, Paula woke me to say the lights of the city were out and it was very quiet. The city going black could have been because of a power failure. The city going quiet was an entirely different matter. I had just read Peter Enahoro's book *How to Be a Nigerian*, in which he quips: "On the sixth day, He created the Nigerian and there was peace. But on the seventh day while God rested, the Nigerian invented noise."[1] Paula said, "I don't like this. Fill the bathtub with water." I replied, "Don't be silly. Go to sleep." A minute later, the first practice mortar shells were launched and we heard machine gun firing. I filled the bathtub with water.

In April, the U.S. Embassy issued the instruction that American women and children had to evacuate from Eastern Nigeria because of the heightened threat of military action. Evacuation flights out of Port Harcourt had been arranged for a Sunday. Missionary families streamed into Enugu on their way to Port Harcourt. On the Friday evening before, I was presented with a large stack of yellow vaccination booklets by the missionary families who had helped during the outbreak in Ogoja the previous December. They had all been vaccinated too, but updating their international vaccination certificates had not seemed a priority at the time. Now they would require proof of vaccination for entry into the United States. This was routine and seemed to pose no special problem. Dr. Anezanwu had a vaccination stamp to certify the vaccinations.

The following morning, Saturday, I took the fifty or so certificates to the Ministry of Health to be stamped, only to learn that Dr. Anezanwu was traveling and would not be back until Monday. I knew where he kept the stamp because the smallpox team members had used it on previous occasions with his permission, so I entered his office by a back door. To my complete surprise, I found his desk locked. Waiting until he returned on Monday was clearly not an option. With some chagrin, I managed to get the drawer open with a pocket knife, but in the process I accidentally broke the lock. I decided that on Monday I would simply explain what had happened and why and have the lock repaired. I stamped the certificates and returned them to those who would be traveling the next day.

Sunday was a difficult day. Paula, David, and Michael were scheduled to be on one of the flights out of Port Harcourt too. The roads were crowded. People could take with them only what fit into a single suitcase. Families were emotional as they approached the moment of being split apart. It was especially heart-rending when people of the region stopped us for an explanation. Why were we leaving? And if we felt in danger, should they worry about their own safety? They had no option of leaving. The airport in Port Harcourt was chaotic as soldiers searched through every suitcase before approving it for travel. On the planes, children would be sitting on adults' laps to maximize the number of people flying out.

Tempers were short. One husband objected when his wife was asked to open her suitcase a second time, saying that it had already been searched. The soldier had the man removed, under guard, to an adjoining room. Only then did the wife realize that her husband had the key to the suitcase. She asked me to see if I could get the key. As I reached the door of the room, I heard the husband asking if he could go out to give the key to his wife. "No," was the answer. "What would you do if I walked over, gave her the key, and walked right back to this room?" "Shoot you," the guard replied. Testing the guard, the man stood up—and the guard cocked and leveled his gun. The husband sat down.

I asked the guard, "Could the two of us keep him from getting into even more trouble? Could he give you the key, you give it to me, and I will give it to his wife?" The guard agreed, and tension was reduced, but the husband was not given an opportunity to say good-bye.

The heavily loaded DC-6s finally left the ground but seemed to take forever to get above one hundred feet in altitude. It was the beginning of hard traveling for the women and children; they would be flying from Port Harcourt to Lagos, then to Dakar, Puerto Rico, and finally New York. It was also a depressing moment for the men who remained behind. Dave, Paul, and I drove back to Enugu to continue our work, determined to eliminate smallpox from the region before we ourselves would have to leave.

Arriving at work at the Ministry of Health the next morning, I was surprised to see police and detectives throughout the building. My secretary told me that someone had broken into Dr. Anezanwu's desk over the weekend and they were getting ready to fingerprint all of the workers. With my recent arrest seared into my mind, I decided this was not the best moment to explain to the ministry what had happened. I told my secretary I would be at the hospital if he needed me. When I went to work the next morning, I heard that the investigators were unable to solve the mystery.

THE LAST OUTBREAK IN EASTERN NIGERIA

Less than six months into using the surveillance/containment strategy, the Enugu team had an opportunity to share what we were discovering with the rest of the West and Central Africa program. The CDC in Atlanta called a meeting in Accra, Ghana, in the first week of July 1967 for all the CDC personnel involved in the West and Central African eradication program. The purpose of the meeting was to see how people were settling in and to identify tactics that were working and could be replicated. Our Enugu team worked hard in our spare moments preparing a presentation. We developed maps that detailed the epidemiology of smallpox in previous years in Eastern Nigeria and summarized the approach we had taken, with graphs and charts showing the preliminary results. Even as we got ready to leave for the Accra meeting, only a single known outbreak remained in the entire Eastern Region, and containment teams were working on it.

Only at the meeting did we realize that while we reported that we had all but eliminated smallpox from our program area, many of the other West African programs were still getting organized. This difference in timing was partly due to political and logistical problems, since USAID negotiated and signed a separate agreement with each of the twenty countries. In some cases, these negotiations required many months. For some attendees, our change in strategy was of little importance because they were not yet far enough along to consider the program in depth. Others, such as Don Millar and Henry Gelfand, who had flown in from Atlanta, were very interested in what we were reporting.

With war brewing, leaving Eastern Nigeria for the meeting was a calculated risk. On May 30, the leaders of Eastern Nigeria had publicly declared the region the Republic of Biafra. However, the American

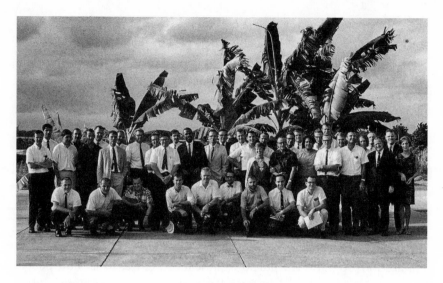

Figure 7. The first cadre of smallpox warriors at a meeting in Accra, Ghana, July 1967

consulate in Enugu had advised us that it would still be a few months before military action began, and we expected to be gone for only a week. Even so, we faced a logistical problem. By this time, there was no official way to cross the border from Biafra into Nigeria and back again. It was common knowledge, though, that people could leave and reenter unofficially at a number of border points. We identified one such a place on the Niger River, had our passports stamped by the Biafrans, hired a large canoe to take us across the river, and then had our passports stamped by Nigerians on the other side. We intended to do the reverse on our return. We then hired a taxi to take us to Lagos, and from there we flew to Accra.

As it turned out, war broke out while we were in Accra. We could not go back to the Eastern Region. Thompson and Lichfield returned to Atlanta. I returned to Nigeria and was assigned by the CDC office in Lagos to work in Northern Nigeria. However, because I had been working in the Eastern Region when the war started, I was arrested almost immediately, held under house arrest for four days at the home of a smallpox worker in Kaduna, and then told to leave the country. I returned to the United States and worked at the CDC on contract for Don Millar, assisting with the African smallpox eradication program from the States while we waited for the end of what we thought would be a short civil war.

It was not until September 1968 that Paula and our two boys and I finally returned to Nigeria, this time to Lagos. I was hired by the International Committee of the Red Cross as a deputy field officer under the supervision of Dr. Wolfgang Bulle, my church program supervisor, who had been hired as the field commander. He asked me to develop surveillance systems detailing refugee movements, food acquisition and use, and disease problems in the refugee camps in areas reclaimed by the federal army. Workers detailed by CDC maintained this program over the next fifteen months.

After Enugu fell to federal forces, I had the opportunity to revisit our flat in Enugu. The military arranged for a police officer to accompany me. The flat was barren except for six inches of files covering the floor. With the police officer standing guard, I began to sort through the papers to see if anything should be salvaged. Coming across a picture, I handed it to the police officer and said, "This is my family." Soon he placed his gun against the wall and got on his knees and began to straighten papers. He said that he had been present at the fall of Enugu and that our flat had been ransacked by federal troops. He apologized for what had happened to our belongings. The juxtaposition of fierceness and tenderness in this man's behavior characterized many interactions during this time of civil war.

It had been more than a year since any of us on the CDC smallpox team had been in Enugu, and during that time we had no way of finding out whether that last outbreak had been contained or not. It was a great moment when we finally discovered that the containment had been successful and stopped transmission for the entire region. Indeed, the Eastern Region had had no reported cases of smallpox during the two and a half years of fighting. For a few suspected cases of smallpox, it was possible to get specimens from these patients to the laboratory; analysis showed the rashes were due to vaccinia and not smallpox; the strain of vaccinia was the same as that in the smallpox vaccine being used in the area.

If we had known how small the window of opportunity would be when we embarked on the new strategy, we undoubtedly would have taken a more aggressive approach—mounting more containment teams, increasing the number of vaccinations for each outbreak. Yet proceeding as we did turned out to be enough.

ERADICATION ESCALATION IN WEST AND CENTRAL AFRICA

In 1967, as eradication efforts expanded not only in the twenty African countries but also to other parts of the world, approximately 130,000 cases of smallpox were reported to WHO. Given the estimated ratio of reported cases to actual cases, WHO later estimated that the number was actually in the millions. Of the forty-four countries that reported cases that year, smallpox was considered endemic in thirty-three of them; that is, continued smallpox transmission did not depend on importations from other countries. These included Brazil, Sub-Saharan Africa, Indonesia, and especially the area stretching from Afghanistan eastward through Pakistan, India, and Nepal to Bangladesh.

After the success of the surveillance/containment approach in Eastern Nigeria in 1967, Don Millar became an enthusiastic advocate of the strategy. While I was at the CDC, he and I developed an effort code-named Eradication Escalation for introducing the strategy throughout the West and Central African program. This effort would include identifying and containing chains of transmission during the seasonal low period of smallpox transmission, since every chain broken during the low period meant far fewer cases to deal with during the following high season.

The approach caught on at different rates and to varying degrees in different countries. For one thing, the original agreement between each country and USAID called for a combined measles and smallpox vaccination program. Since administering the measles vaccine to every child between six months and six years of age required a mass vaccination approach, adopting the surveillance/containment strategy meant managing two very different methodologies at the same time. In some countries the CDC teams were able to do this. In Dahomey (now Benin), twelve independent smallpox teams on motorcycles—smallpox outbreak chasers, if you will—traveled the country responding to outbreaks and containing them while others were doing mass vaccinations.

Moreover, the CDC staff had been trained to apply mass vaccination as the primary strategy. The idea of making surveillance/containment the primary strategy felt too risky and counterintuitive to some, while others embraced it. In Sierra Leone, for instance, which had some of the highest smallpox rates in the world, the director of the program, Donald Hopkins, used surveillance/containment with great success.

Once a geographical area began the surveillance/containment strategy, smallpox rarely persisted there for more than twelve to fifteen months. Eventually, all twenty countries in the CDC program made use of this approach, and smallpox disappeared from each one. Nigeria was the most daunting challenge because of its large population—which equaled that of all the other nineteen countries combined. Stan Foster, head of the Nigerian program, was successful to varying degrees in getting the strategy adopted in the Northern, Western, and Midwest regions. Nigeria recorded its final case of smallpox in May 1970.

West and Central Africa was expected to be the most challenging region of the world for smallpox eradication, yet it became the first geographical area in the WHO program to become free of smallpox. The program goal had been to eliminate smallpox within five years. The last case was reported from Nigeria only three years and six months after the program's start—and the program was under budget. Former U.S. surgeon general Julius Richmond, commenting on the miracle of smallpox eradication in West Africa in such a short time, said that the smallpox workers sent by CDC were "simply too young to realize they couldn't do it." In fact, they were well chosen for the job, people who proved they could meet any problem—difficulties with vehicles, jet injectors, camels, communications, or government officials—with high spirits and humor. And they were armed with an appropriate tool for the task.

However, WHO still took a cautious stance. In 1968, the WHO Expert Committee report, while accepting the importance of both strategies, was not prepared to accept surveillance/containment as the *primary* strategy in highly endemic situations. The report states,

> The objective of the smallpox eradication programme is achieved by reducing the prevalence of smallpox to the point where transmission of the disease is terminated. Normally, as a first step, this requires systematic mass vaccination with potent freeze-dried vaccine to reduce the prevalence of disease. Simultaneously, however, a case-detection and reporting system should be established or improved to permit prompt application of containment measures, thereby interrupting further transmission. Both these aspects of the eradication programme must receive adequate attention but perhaps greater weight should be given to mass vaccination in highly endemic, poorly vaccinated areas, shifting the emphasis to case detection and reporting as endemic disease declines and a more satisfactory state of herd immunity is achieved.[2]

Attitudes were changing by 1968, but the herd immunity strategy still drove WHO's thinking.

The twenty-country program yielded several new insights into the epidemiology of smallpox, each of which helped to refine the eradication strategy. Both folklore and textbooks described smallpox as a disease of rapid transmission. In fact, the CDC workers discovered that the virus spread with more difficulty than expected, often requiring multiple incubation periods even within one household or compound. The virus's tenacity in continuing to infect new generations within a household was confused with high transmissibility, which explains its false reputation as a highly contagious disease. This understanding of the epidemiology meant that the natural progression of an outbreak could indeed be interrupted.[3]

We also observed the accumulated wisdom of countless generations who had faced the disease. During an outbreak temporary structures were constructed outside a village to house patients. Persons who had recovered from smallpox were in charge of bringing food to the patients and caring for them. It was common knowledge that having had the disease itself provided solid immunity. Experience also showed that few people who had a visible smallpox vaccination scar got smallpox, and that cases were extremely rare in persons with a history of a second vaccination.

Gradually, we also discovered that the incubation period for vaccinia virus, the virus used in vaccine, was slightly shorter than the incubation period for the smallpox virus itself. Therefore, vaccinating a person on the day of exposure to smallpox could prevent the disease. Indeed, we eventually learned that vaccination even several days after exposure could prevent or at least reduce the severity of the disease. In the race between the two viruses, the vaccine virus could win.

THE SURVEILLANCE/CONTAINMENT STRATEGY: NEW OR NOT NEW?

Was the surveillance/containment strategy that was proving so effective with smallpox new or not new? The two basic parts of the strategy were not new. Surveillance is the basis for all disease control programs at CDC and elsewhere in the world. One could not work at CDC without deeply internalizing the idea that disease control requires accurate knowledge about the disease and its environment and that this knowledge is obtained through surveillance systems. Response, or control, was based on surveillance findings.

The global smallpox program was designed to reduce smallpox virus transmission by means of mass vaccination to a point where attention could be placed on individual outbreaks and chains of transmission. The WHO program, from the beginning, envisioned surveillance and containment as the follow-on strategy after mass vaccination. Henry Gelfand and D. A. Henderson describe the original strategy for the West Africa program in a 1966 article in the *Journal of International Health*. They state that the goal of the program "being eradication, an attempt will be made to vaccinate the entire population, regardless of age or previous vaccination status, in as short a time as possible"—in other words, to do mass vaccination. They go on to say that this will probably take two or three years. Because 100 percent coverage is unrealistic, "a second mass cycle of vaccination will probably be carried out within the 5-year lifetime of the program." In addition, they say that because disease surveillance is "grossly incomplete," the "epidemiologists will be intimately concerned with the mobilization of every available reporting source . . . so that no case of smallpox will go unreported and uninvestigated." The idea was to pinpoint areas of transmission not eliminated by mass vaccination. Finally, they list what they regard as the more important new elements of the program. These included a regional approach, the use of lyophilized vaccine and jet injectors, a systematic assessment and surveillance program, and adequate resources.[4]

The handbook for all CDC workers in the program, titled *West and Central African Smallpox Eradication/Measles Control Program: Manual of Operations*, clearly sets out the program's expectations: to develop a mass vaccination program and to complete the program within three years, before immunity could wane:

> Since the target with respect to smallpox is eradication, a finite goal, and since this involves a careful systematic vaccination of all ages and segments of the population, operational procedures and techniques focus principally on smallpox vaccination . . . smallpox eradication will be realized by successfully reducing, through vaccination, the number of susceptibles in the West African population to the point where it is impossible for the disease to sustain itself in a continuous chain of transmission.
>
> Since the objective of the vaccination campaign is to induce a high level of immunity in the population . . . [and since] after three years, the proportion of persons with full immunity falls gradually and "breakthroughs" become more frequent . . . obtaining total coverage in three years requires realistic planning.[5]

In fact, the manual included a warning to not let outbreak containment divert efforts from the mass campaign during the three years. "The need may occasionally arise for a rapid vaccination effort in an area to control an outbreak. In pre-planning, provision should be made for handling these situations. For completion of the attack phase on schedule, the time table drawn up for area coverage should be reasonably strictly followed. If vaccination teams are frequently forced to disrupt their activities to perform mopping up or 'fire fighting' operations, great damage will be done to the orderly progress of the campaign."[6]

Surveillance/containment approaches were not new to the CDC team. Vaccinating those at highest risk of exposure makes logical sense and had been used frequently. Indeed, it was endorsed by a royal commission in England as early as the 1890s. Surveillance/containment was also written into plans for the containment of a possible smallpox importation in various cities (such as New York) and had been used for outbreak control in many countries, especially importations of smallpox into Europe in the twentieth century. As already mentioned, it was also the follow-on plan in the WHO program after mass vaccination had reduced the intensity of transmission. This was the reason for developing the surveillance system for identifying all cases of smallpox. While surveillance/containment was the logical follow-on to mass vaccination, it was always seen in a secondary role, never as the primary strategy and certainly not as a substitute for mass vaccination.

After the positive results in Ogoja province (and later in the entire Eastern Region of Nigeria), however, surveillance and containment began to be seen as the *primary* strategy for smallpox eradication. This had not been presented as an option in our training before we left for Africa. The lessons learned in the outbreak in Ogoja province led eventually to the abandonment of mass vaccination as the primary strategy in other countries and finally in all countries as eradication activities rapidly accelerated. When surveillance and containment are made the primary strategy, mass vaccination can be dropped totally. In fact, it becomes a wasted effort.

In retrospect, it is easy to see why surveillance and containment worked so well for this particular disease. The presence of the virus was easy to detect, since almost everyone infected developed lesions, mostly on the face and extremities, where they were easily seen. Moreover, most people who acquired the virus became so severely ill that it stopped their movement. Family, friends, and community members were likely to be aware of cases. Even if a patient remained undetected from the first day of the rash, the chain of transmission didn't remain hidden for long. Even if only a single person was infected during each incubation period, which is two or three weeks, only twenty persons were needed to keep a single chain of transmission intact for a year. If any one of those twenty people failed to pass the virus on, the chain was broken. In fact, in most cases, an annual chain involved hundreds of people, making the virus easy to find.

Not only did the virus have difficulty remaining incognito during the illness, it also left a trail after the fact. Pockmarks, especially on the face, told the story of the virus's visit. Surveys of a village quickly revealed the last time the virus was active in the community, based on the age of the youngest people showing scars. The bottom line is that unlike many other viruses, smallpox virus simply could not hide. It left too many clues.

The ease of identifying the smallpox virus is highlighted by an incident in November 1971. Smallpox workers at the CDC in Atlanta watching the nightly news happened to see a report about refugees leaving Bangladesh, bound for India. One of the refugees in the film clip appeared to have smallpox. The Atlanta observers called the report in to WHO in Geneva. The WHO alerted officials in India, who alerted local workers, and the following day the outbreak was found and contained.

Surveillance and containment also works particularly well for smallpox because the virus is so specialized. It can only commandeer human cells. Over the centuries it must have tried repeatedly to adapt to other species, but without success. The smallpox virus must find a new, susceptible host within weeks of initiating disease in a person or it will die. The virus also dies quickly outside the human body unless it is kept in freezing conditions. It turned out that a perimeter containing no susceptible people needed to extend for only a half-dozen feet from the person with smallpox to be effective. Therefore, once the virus was located, vaccinators could concentrate their efforts on vaccinating anyone who might have come within that perimeter. It was necessary, of course, to prevent the virus from traveling out of that protective bubble on contaminated clothes—just as firefighters must prevent a fire from crossing a fire line.

Although the surveillance/containment method worked exceedingly well for smallpox, this does not mean it would work as effectively for other diseases. The smallpox eradication story contains many lessons, but giving up mass vaccination as a methodology for other diseases is not one of them. Rather, the lesson is that every problem has to be considered individually.

Our experience in Eastern Nigeria and then in West and Central Africa was compelling. Surveillance/containment was eventually used as the primary strategy in all areas of the world in the smallpox eradication effort. It would be refined and tested to the utmost and would provide its most dramatic results seven years in the future, in the state of Bihar, India. But it started that night in Ogoja province during a problem-solving discussion about inadequate supplies.

PART TWO India

MEETING THE CHALLENGE OF ERADICATION

SIX

Under the Rule of Variola

As the new decade began, the win column in the global effort to eradicate smallpox started to lengthen. In January 1971, nine months after the last smallpox case in West and Central Africa, Brazil reported its final case. Three months later, Indonesia became free of smallpox. By the end of the year, only nine countries still had continuous smallpox transmission. In July 1972, Afghanistan became smallpox free.

Yet even as the number of countries with smallpox was declining, progress was disappointing in the four smallpox-endemic countries of South Asia: Bangladesh, India, Nepal, and Pakistan. In India, a new mass vaccination campaign, the fourth within ten years, was having little impact. There was strong feeling both inside and outside the country that smallpox in India was different, that success in other places simply underscored the problem. Even experienced public health workers, including some with extensive experience in the Africa smallpox program, came away frustrated, concluding that the problems of smallpox in India could not be approached in the same way as elsewhere. In India, it seemed, smallpox was inevitable.

By this time I was back in Atlanta, working at the CDC as director of the smallpox program. Dr. David J. Sencer, then director of CDC, had a passion for getting smallpox eradicated. He was a bright, dedicated physician who took delight in solving problems.

The CDC had remained involved in the WHO global program even after eradication was accomplished in West and Central Africa. At the beginning of the program, Leo Morris was assigned to work in Brazil, and then a flood of CDC people were assigned around the world. Most were assigned through WHO, but a few were assigned directly on a bilateral basis. CDC staff traveled frequently in response to WHO requests, evaluating programs and attending WHO-sponsored meetings. The working relationship between CDC and WHO was so close that any jurisdictional issues or turf problems could be negotiated. The combined heft of the two agencies was often important, since public health officials looked to the CDC on questions of science but expected consultants to come with a WHO stamp of approval.

I found that the ideal position was to be seconded, that is, loaned, by CDC to WHO for work in the field. I used my WHO position when working with administrative or political staff and my CDC position when working with scientific staff. Most work straddled both areas. Because of my experience with the surveillance/containment methodology, I was often asked to present at WHO meetings in various parts of the world.

The surveillance and containment method had been promoted at every global smallpox meeting since the regional meeting in Accra in July 1967. The idea was strongly pushed in letters from WHO/Geneva to the WHO regional office in New Delhi. However, surveillance and containment as the primary strategy was simply not imagined in India. Many seriously doubted that smallpox transmission could be interrupted in high population density areas where smallpox was endemic. Henry Gelfand, for instance, a longtime CDC public health worker, had been part of an evaluation of smallpox in India that recommended virtually 100 percent vaccination coverage as the only way to interrupt smallpox transmission in that country.

In a May 2, 1969, letter to Don Millar, then chief of the smallpox program at CDC, Gelfand voiced his doubts that the method that had been so successful in Africa would be applicable in South Asia:

> It is a remarkable document, and its exposition and description of "Eradication Escalation" will make it a landmark in the history of disease eradication. . . .
>
> In a luscious bowl of honey, however, one must look out for the rare fly that may be trapped and spoil the dish. I do have a tiny complaint, because I well know how some people in this world can quote out of context to select a point which will serve their own self interest or justify their own complacency. In about the middle of page 6 this sentence appears, "This approach (referring to search/investigation/ control) is now considered of equal and, under certain circumstances, of *even greater importance* than systematic mass campaign activities." I should rather see the underlining applied to a different phrase as follows, "This approach is now considered of equal and, *under certain circumstances*, of even greater importance than systematic mass campaign activities."
>
> I am sure that you had in mind the unusual nature of the circumstances pertaining in the West African program in the fall of last year: the unusually high ratio of epidemiologists to population, the caliber of the epidemiologists, the availability of special surveillance/control teams, the non-interruption of intensive and concurrent mass vaccination activities. Deliberately or stupidly misinterpreted, the emphasis given in the original sentence could be used to justify fruitless and inefficient epidemic chasing in India and Pakistan. Please don't give them the chance.[1]

The power of surveillance/containment to stop transmission had been demonstrated in 1968 and 1969 in the South Indian state of Tamil Nadu in a program directed by Dr. A. R. Rao, following the reports from West Africa in 1967. However, Rao introduced surveillance/containment after mass vaccination had already reduced smallpox to a few hundred cases. In essence, he had simply confirmed the WHO's original recommendation of using mass vaccination first, followed by surveillance and containment as a secondary strategy. It was a success for Tamil Nadu but did not actually test surveillance/containment as a primary strategy in an area of high population density.[2]

In the spring of 1973, a breakthrough in thinking occurred in India. During the seasonal high-transmission period, which runs from January through May or June, major outbreaks were discovered in a district in South India believed to be free of smallpox. The health staff mobilized to do a house-to-house search to determine the extent of the epidemic. Two weeks of preparation led to a ten-day search, which a later assessment found to be surprisingly complete. The searchers discovered numerous unreported outbreaks, which were rapidly contained. The district became free of smallpox in a matter of weeks.

This experience demonstrated that India's large health staff could readily be mobilized for search and containment activities. More importantly, it showed that the smallpox virus in India played by international rules.

Soon after this, Dave Sencer told me that D. A. Henderson at WHO Geneva wanted to assign me to India as a consultant to the WHO regional office in New Delhi to help them apply the surveillance/containment strategy to smallpox-endemic South Asia. The first step was to visit India and meet with the Indian and WHO staff to determine their interest in having me join their program.

My coworkers at the CDC advised me not to go unless I had a solid contract with WHO and India that spelled out what would be provided and what my authority would be. Since I had no idea what the job would require, I found it impossible to specify details. In the end, there was no contract. As the eradication effort progressed, I was very happy that I had gone without preconditions. No one could have predicted the scope of the challenges and how job descriptions would morph dramatically to meet the needs of the moment. Almost any prior agreement would have hampered the effort.

In the summer of 1973, I visited New Delhi—my first time back in India since serving with the Peace Corps in 1963. I found that my interest in the country had not diminished. I met Dr. Nicole Grasset, director of smallpox eradication in WHO's Southeast Asia Regional Office (SEARO), and was immediately impressed by her enthusiasm and desire for success. I also met with the staff at the Government of India's Ministry of Health at Nirman Bhavan and at the National Institute of Communicable

Diseases. At their request, I addressed a meeting of state smallpox leaders gathered in New Delhi to plan a national strategy. I was asked to share the West African experience and to inspire the group to embrace the strategy that had worked so well in that setting. I was wearing, under my dress shirt, a T-shirt that said, in large letters, "Smallpox Zero." At the high point of my talk I said that we would gird for this historic battle and settle for nothing less than . . . I undid my necktie and unbuttoned and pulled my shirt open so the audience could read "Smallpox Zero." There was no reaction!

There was nothing to do but bring my talk to an anticlimactic close as I rebuttoned my shirt. It was not a great start. A year later, the same closing would have elicited applause and cheering. Timing is everything, and I was a year off.

In consultation with my family, I made the decision to go to India to work under Dr. Grasset as a CDC consultant. I arranged to spend an additional week in New Delhi, preparing for our move. However, I became so involved in smallpox discussions that in the end I had only the last day of my visit to make personal arrangements. With a great deal of help, a week's worth of activity was accomplished in that whirlwind day—a harbinger of what was possible in India.

I rented a ground-floor flat in Maharani Bagh, New Delhi, that came without furniture but would be fixed up, painted, and ready for our arrival in August. I arranged for air-conditioning units to be installed in the bedrooms. I went to two different specialty offices, where I rented furniture and a refrigerator. After reviewing recommendations by former WHO workers, I secured the services of a cook, N. Joseph, who in turn agreed to arrange for a gardener and a night watchman. I then opened a bank account, registered the children for school, and signed an agreement for an Indian-made car and a driver. I interviewed several drivers, as I wanted someone who was slow and careful so I could feel secure about our children. In Jit Singh I found the perfect person. I ended the day exhausted but energized, able to depart happily for the airport that night to return to Atlanta.

Even living in Africa did not adequately prepare us for the adventure of life in India. During the twenty months we were there, the children never lost their fascination with it. The day after we arrived, Paula, myself, and our three boys, David, Michael, and three-year-old Robert, explored New Delhi in the rented car with Jit Singh as driver. Cows, camels, and bullocks walked in the streets alongside motor scooters, three-wheeler taxis, buses, and foot traffic. Affluent shaded residential areas stood in stark contrast to slum areas with houses made of discarded materials. We saw brightly colored flowers, saris in every color, and even colorful old buildings, such as the Red Fort. Stores of all kinds bore witness to the spirit of entrepreneurship and the thriving marketplace. Michael, now age seven, had his nose pressed to the window. Suddenly he turned and said, "This is the second best day in my whole life." Surprised, I asked him, "What was the first best day?" He said, "Yesterday."

SMALLPOX IN INDIA'S HISTORY

An outsider should approach everything about India, including its history, ready to put preconceptions aside. India is overwhelming in its scope and confusing in its detail, as well as in the lessons it provides. Its history abounds with items never taught in U.S. schools, such as the efficiency of Chandragupta, who recaptured India from the Macedonian authority left by Alexander the Great to form the most powerful government in the world at that time. His organizational skills were impressive: he ordered his day into sixteen 90-minute periods. We hear little about the ruler Ashoka, who, after developing a reputation for cruelty, abruptly changed and based his government on the golden rule. We generally are not exposed to the decency of Krishna Raya, a contemporary of Henry VIII; the wisdom of Akbar, who created the most powerful empire of the time; or the paradox of Shah Jehan, who left a trail of ruthlessness and artistic beauty.

The religious, political, and artistic histories of India are matched by its scientific contributions. Astronomy and mathematics come immediately to mind. India is credited with inventing the zero. Indian medical sciences were describing the circulation of the blood before the time of

Harvey, and offered a medical creed before Hippocrates. Nalanda, a red-bricked university whose ruins are in Bihar state, flourished for more than a millennium before Cambridge was even founded.

The history of smallpox in India is intertwined in the subcontinent's history and is no less ancient and complex. Smallpox was very likely present in India for a very long time, although evidence dating before the sixteenth century is circumstantial and mainly found in Hindu myths and Brahmin traditions. J. Z. Holwell, in his eighteenth-century *Account of the Manner of Inoculating for the Smallpox in the East Indies*, comments that the Brahmin caste maintained traditions concerning smallpox from time immemorial.[3] Smallpox was probably known in India at the time of Ramses V.[4] The *Atharva Veda*, an ancient Hindu scripture dated to the twelfth to tenth century B.C.E., describes the worship of a deity whose protection was invoked on the outbreak of this disease. It also describes rituals and prayers to be done by Brahmins at the time of inoculation, or variolation, with smallpox.[5]

Many cultures have believed that angry deities get their revenge by causing death and disease in humans. In India, smallpox was believed to be caused by Sitala-Mata, or Devi, the goddess responsible for pustular diseases.[6] The strength of this belief is evident in historical documents. For example, Hindu residents of Kanpur wrote an appeal when the colonial government decided to make vaccination compulsory in 1888: "The major portion of our community believes that small-pox is the direct expression of the wrath of the Goddess Bhawani or Shitala. It is not a malady that can be cured by medicine, and any attempt to check its progress will only enrage the Goddess, who is otherwise pacified by prayers and simple diet. The belief is founded on sacred texts . . . and . . . we believe that our just Government will not offend the religious feelings of its loyal subjects."[7]

The goddess was depicted in different forms and bears different names in different parts of the country. Because the annual increase in cases occurred in the springtime, in the eastern and northeastern regions the disease was called *basonto* (relating to the spring) or *guti basonto* (nodules appearing in the spring). In southern India, it was known as *peria ammai* or *doddamma* (big goddess) or *vaisuri noi* (disease with eruptions).

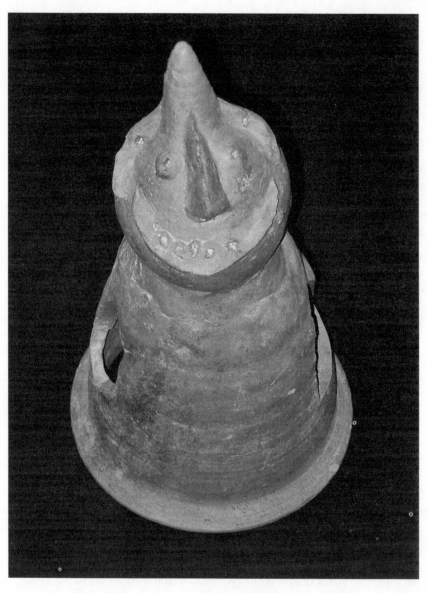

Figure 8. A village smallpox goddess (far less elaborate than was typical)

As India's population density increased through the centuries, smallpox may have become an almost universal disease, a rite of passage, truly democratic in its disregard for caste or economic status. Cities were probably its major focus, especially during the low-transmission time of the year, during the monsoons. As travel increased again after the monsoons, the virus would be seeded to rural areas through commerce and family visits.

In India, as in Africa, variolation evidently existed for centuries, which meant that, religious beliefs notwithstanding, Indian society had long been aware that a simple operation could protect against smallpox. Holwell describes how a group of Brahmins traveled on a circuit to provide inoculations before the seasonal upswing of smallpox. They followed careful protocols, requiring an entire village to agree to inoculation before they would begin, and asking the village to remain isolated from other villages until the lesions had healed. Apparently the results were so good that the demand for variolation soon exceeded the Brahmin ability to respond. This led to an increase in the price charged for the procedure. The marketplace took over, less careful operators proliferated, entire villages were no longer inoculated at the same time, and outbreaks of smallpox resulted.[8] During the early days of vaccination, variolators often resisted vaccination because it competed with their livelihood, although some readily transferred their skills and became vaccinators.

While there is no question that smallpox had a long history in India, its full impact is less clear. Early records on smallpox mortality are simply unavailable. During the colonial period, the British attempted to collect data systematically, but their statistics are open to interpretation. We know, for example, that seventy-five years after Jenner's first vaccination in 1796, India recorded nearly two hundred thousand deaths in a single year. However, in that time of incomplete record keeping, the actual number had to be larger.

In 1883, in the single state of Uttar Pradesh, over 138,000 deaths were recorded; over 202,000 were recorded the following year. As the population of the state was then estimated at 5 million, these figures indicate that about 7 percent of the population of Uttar Pradesh died of smallpox during those two years. If mortality rates were about one-third, as they were in the twentieth century, it would appear that over 20 percent of the population of Uttar Pradesh acquired smallpox during that two-year span.[9] This is without adjusting the numbers to allow for incomplete records.

It is easier to get accurate records for royal families. The history of the Tipparah royal family reveals that between the fifteenth and eighteenth centuries, five of the sixteen maharajas died of smallpox. Again using a mortality rate of about one-third, this suggests that all sixteen may have actually acquired the disease.[10]

EARLY VACCINATION EFFORTS

Vaccination efforts in India began almost immediately after Jenner's discovery in 1796. In 1799, Jenner himself shipped copies of his paper and a quantity of cowpox material on the East India ship *The Queen*, but the ship was wrecked before reaching India.[11] The vaccine finally made it to India three years later, after vaccination was successfully established in Constantinople and Baghdad. This strain of vaccine can be traced back to Jean de Carro from Vienna and from him to Luigi Sacco, who acquired it in 1800 from a herd of Swiss cows at a county fair near the border between Italy and Switzerland.[12] Therefore, in the final analysis, it was Jenner's idea but not his vaccine that started the program in India.

Spread of vaccine throughout the country was not simple. When attempts to ship dried cowpox material on cotton threads proved unsuccessful, the decision was made to deliver the virus from place to place through a series of children. As lesions developed in their skin, they in turn became the donor of virus to the next susceptible child, in this way maintaining a chain of viable cowpox virus propagated in human lymph. In Bombay, on June 14, 1802, Dr. Helenus Scott successfully vaccinated the first child, a three-year-old girl, Anna Dusthall. From this child the vaccine virus spread outward from Bombay. Accounts exist that track its spread. For example, spreading the virus from Madras to Calcutta required five children and five weeks. On October 10, 1802,

Dr. James Anderson vaccinated a thirteen-year-old boy, John Cresswell, using material from the vaccination of an Indian child. With Cresswell, Dr. Anderson boarded the ship *Hunter*. Twelve days later, Anderson vaccinated a girl using material from Cresswell's lesion. On November 2, the fourth child, a boy, was vaccinated by using material from the girl's lesion, and on November 12, a fifth child, a boy by the name of Charles Norton, was vaccinated. Norton became the source of vaccine for Calcutta when the ship arrived on November 17.[13]

British workers in India not only were some of the first to be vaccinated, but also were among the first to show their gratitude to Jenner. In May 1806, when the benefits of vaccination were still being argued in England, there was no confusion in the message sent along with a gift of £4,000 (a huge sum in those days) to Jenner from "the principal inhabitants of Calcutta and its dependencies as a testimonial of their gratitude for the benefits which this Settlement, in common with the rest of mankind, has derived from his inestimable discovery of a preventive of the smallpox." The example of Calcutta was quickly followed by gifts from Bombay and Madras.[14]

As vaccination activities spread through the country, great inequities developed. Early operations were primarily restricted to easily accessible urban areas, which limited the impact of the vaccination effort. This was to be the lament for the next 150 years. Since evaluation was based on the number of vaccinations, not the percentage of the population protected, vaccinators could fulfill their assignment by returning to easily reached groups, such as schoolchildren in urban areas, to give them repeat vaccinations. Vaccination activities were extended to villages only in response to specific reports of smallpox cases and deaths.

Some groups resisted vaccination, sometimes for religious reasons, sometimes because of their distrust of the government. R. W. Hunter noted in 1876 that the Biharis were particularly reluctant to be vaccinated.[15] This was still the case one hundred years later, and Bihar was the last state in India where smallpox transmission was interrupted. Some areas of the country were late to be served. Hopkins reports that vaccination did not reach Kashmir until 1894. And, while the rich and the educated are often at the head of the line to receive health services, vaccinators would sometimes vaccinate lower caste persons first in order to demonstrate that the procedure was safe.[16]

Widespread vaccination requires a dependable source of vaccine. For three decades, the vaccine supply in India could be traced to the propagation of the virus from that first vaccination of Anna Dusthall in Bombay. In 1832, however, Dr. McPherson of Moorshedabad (Murshidabad) reported the discovery of cowpox in Indian cattle, and with this he developed a new source for vaccine. This India-grown lymph was believed superior and it was distributed widely, "where it was speedily mixed with that previously in use."[17]

A dizzying array of vaccination procedures were used in nineteenth-century India. Some vaccinations were given from person to person. Some vaccinators took inoculated calves with them to the site of vaccinations and applied the lymph directly from calf to human. Experiments were even attempted using goats and donkeys as vectors for the vaccine. Techniques for applying vaccine also varied, ranging from minor abrasions of the skin to deep incisions into which the material was placed. Vaccination locations varied from sites on the arm that would be familiar today to "the inner side at the bend of the elbow" or "the base of the right thumb in males and the left in females."[18] Because the vaccinia virus was viable only for a period of days, attempts were made to store it in vials or ampules with a wide variety of preservatives.

It is often thought that British colonial administrators imposed a vaccination program across India that was stymied by the people's resistance to it. Hopkins relates a story of Indian priests at Benares who told of an old prophecy that India would expel the British through the leadership of a black child with white blood. Vaccination, the priests charged, was how the English intended to find that child to kill him.[19]

However, an exhaustive study of the colonial records suggests that, at least in the nineteenth century, the program was largely hampered by technical difficulties.[20] These included the lack of a reliable vaccine (which undermined confidence in the program when people were vaccinated and later got smallpox), the problems of getting calf or human lymph to the area for vaccination, and the painful procedures used to introduce the virus. The program was also slowed by official discord, such as the constant tension between the desire to make local areas responsible for their own protection and reluctance at the central level to release control, the deliberate sabotage of the program by persons who were not convinced it was efficacious, and the pervasive foibles of those jockeying for power.

By 1898, some of the technical difficulties had been solved. Bovine lymph had largely replaced the use of human lymph in all provinces. Vaccinations were conducted either directly from calf to arm or with lymph preserved in tubes, either alone or mixed with glycerin, lanolin, or Vaseline. The State Vaccine Institute in Patwadangar (Uttar Pradesh) was established in 1904, and soon most provinces had a central vaccine depot for the manufacture of animal-derived vaccine.

The British government required that records be kept on smallpox rates, vaccination rates, and program efforts. A summary of countless pages of depressing statistics suggests that more than half a century after the introduction of the smallpox vaccine, the disease continued its relentless decimation of humanity in India. The effect of vaccine could be shown in specific areas, but for various reasons the disease was more than a match for the best efforts of health authorities on a national level.

In a 1909 publication, S. P. James attempted to show the vaccine's effectiveness by charting the decline of smallpox, over ten-year periods, in the provinces of Bombay, the Punjab, and the United Provinces of Agra, Oudh, and Berar, an area he called "well-vaccinated British India."[21] The area had a recorded population of 137 million in the 1901 census. While the decline is obvious, the limited impact of almost a century of preventive efforts is just as evident. Even in the nineteenth century, the science of the day was far ahead of the ability to use it effectively.

To all of this must be added the competition between variolation and vaccination. The results of variolation were known and observable. When a village was variolated, a large percentage of residents would get a mild case of smallpox and the villagers then knew that as a group they were protected. With vaccination, on the other hand, the vaccine was not always reliable, and the occurrence of smallpox cases in previously vaccinated persons was general knowledge. Variolation also had the advantage of religious association. It was both a medical and a religious

---

Table 1   Smallpox deaths in well-vaccinated
British India, 1868–1907

Years	Deaths
1868–77	1,308,737
1878–87	1,242,797
1888–97	747,590
1898–1907	478,843

SOURCE: S. P. James, *Smallpox and Vaccination in
British India* (Calcutta: Thacker, Spink and Co., 1909).

ceremony that included offerings to the goddess of the disease. Even though variolation caused a certain percentage of deaths, many preferred it over vaccination.

In the first half of the twentieth century, smallpox control efforts in India relied heavily on vaccination drives and isolation of patients.[22] However, compulsory programs often simply stiffened any existing resistance, making it harder to get children vaccinated and turning health workers into half-hearted enforcers. A report from Madras indicates that many people were listed as "left the town," which was simply a way of avoiding vaccination. The net impact of compulsory vaccination was an increase in falsification of the records. Attempts to enforce compulsory vaccination resulted in a lot of energy expended for little gain. A 1920s report from the Punjab indicates that 10,500 notices were filed in Lahore against parents who had not vaccinated their children. Only 49 made it to court, which resulted in 18 additional vaccinations. In another report from Jabalpur, in Madhya Pradesh, 1,502 reports for noncompliance led to an additional 5 vaccinations after court trials. Isolation of patients, while effective in theory, also increased the likelihood that families would hide family members with smallpox to avoid being separated from them.

Increasingly, medical authorities concluded that widespread vaccination was required. Yet the disparity in vaccination between urban and rural areas remained a significant obstacle. Rural populations tended to distrust imposed remedies, and rural health workers often resisted the introduction of new vaccines and operating techniques, especially when the additional training was at their own expense. Despite all of the problems, the number of vaccinations increased in the first half of the twentieth century. While mortality statistics for smallpox were as high as 1,000 to 2,000 per million people per year during the three decades between 1870 and 1900, they decreased to highs of 600 per million per year between 1900 and 1925, and finally dropped to about 100 per million per year by 1950. These are high rates for a country to tolerate from a single devastating yet preventable cause. A comparable phenomenon is twentieth-century America's acceptance of lung cancer death rates of 1,300 to 1,500 per million, year after year, because of widespread tobacco use, a situation preventable through education.

Annual vaccinations increased steadily during this period and by the 1940s far exceeded the birth rate, yet 50 percent of smallpox deaths occurred in children under ten years of age. Clearly, the problem was not in the number of vaccinations delivered, but in who was receiving the vaccine. Vaccinators continued to return to easy-to-reach groups year after year, thereby providing superior immunity to some groups while other groups remained totally vulnerable.

In 1946, a report released by the Government of India listed smallpox, cholera, and plague as the three major epidemic diseases and reported that according to the League of Nations, India had the highest incidence of smallpox among all countries for which information was available. The report also noted that the continuing high rates of smallpox deaths in young children revealed the current program's inadequacy, since a single vaccination in infancy could provide almost total protection during childhood.[23]

At the time of its independence, India was saddled with the highest smallpox incidence in the world. During the next quarter century the country would record over four hundred thousand deaths. If Basu is correct in assuming that only 1 percent of actual deaths were reported, the number of deaths was more like 40 million citizens.[24] Would the perception of the power of the Goddess yet win?

NATIONWIDE PROGRAMS

In June 1958, when the World Health Assembly passed the resolution to eradicate smallpox from the world, India responded by forming an expert committee of the Indian Council of Medical Research to suggest the methods to be used in India.[25] The committee called for simultaneous action to be taken in all parts of the country. Noting the shortcomings of previous campaigns, the committee made several recommendations: setting up systems for compulsory registration of vital statistics, with punishments for those responsible for lapses; a Central Infectious Disease Control Act to ensure national uniformity; a central reference laboratory to provide quality control for vaccine production; a national smallpox eradication program to vaccinate the entire population within three years; and pilot projects in each state to develop the necessary procedures. The committee noted the periodicity of epidemics and the seasonal nature of the disease, but did not suggest using seasonality as a means of improving control procedures—even though Brahmin variolators had demonstrated that concentrating their efforts during the periods of low transmission was an effective means of reducing spread during periods of high transmission.

Pilot projects were initiated in each state, and in October 1962, the Government of India launched a nationwide program. Within five months, the entire country was involved in an attack phase, scheduled to extend for two to three years. As in other smallpox eradication plans throughout the world, the objective was mass vaccination, with three years to complete the attack phase and 80 percent coverage during that time—even though there was no scientific evidence showing the efficacy of these three goals. This stage was to be followed with a maintenance phase during which those missed in the attack phase would be vaccinated.

Shortcomings aside, this was the largest commitment the Government of India had ever made to attack smallpox. The logistical and organizational aspects of the campaign were impressive. A central organization was developed in the Directorate General of Health Services to coordinate the program. State organizations and district operating units were developed. Vehicles, vaccine, and other supplies were acquired, and more than thirteen thousand workers were deployed in 152 mobile units. Each mobile unit included 72 vaccinators, 12 sanitary inspectors, 2 health educators, a paramedical assistant, and a medical officer. The Central Government included a budget line of Rs. 68.90 million (about US $8.61 million) to assist state governments, and the USSR provided hundreds of millions of doses of freeze-dried smallpox vaccine.[26]

It soon became obvious that 80 percent coverage was not going to be achieved in two years. Indeed, even if 80 percent coverage had been achieved, it would not have stopped smallpox, given the population density of India. For example, Delhi, while reporting vaccination coverage of 84 percent, was simultaneously in the grip of a smallpox epidemic. Some blamed the epidemic on the fact that so many people were moving into Delhi from all parts of India. But a Delhi-based assessment team demonstrated that for every imported case there were thirty-six local cases. The team also found an unacceptable time lag from the onset of a case until it was reported and outbreak control vaccinations could begin. The euphoria of starting a new program had already run into the brick wall of reality.

Looking for a corrective, the program only ran itself even deeper into the wall. The Delhi assessment committee recommended revising the eradication target from 80 to 100 percent. Given the difficulty of achieving 80 percent coverage in most of the country, this new target could only have lowered morale even further.

In 1964, the Central Council of Health reviewed the progress of the national smallpox eradication program and made the same recommendation: 100 percent vaccination coverage in all sectors of the population. Vaccination figures did increase afterward, but later surveys indicated that this was only because the same easily accessible populations, such as schoolchildren, were being given repeat vaccinations. The same lesson had to be learned repeatedly throughout the world: the number of vaccinations given is a meaningless figure.

A year later, India's National Institute of Communicable Diseases evaluated the smallpox eradication program, examining selected districts around the country.[27] The institute found the following: The reported vaccination figures were much higher than observed figures based on sample surveys of the population. Immunity levels were far lower than anticipated, and primary vaccinations were, in some places, reaching as little as 50 percent of the target population. Take rates varied from 40 to 95 percent, depending on the technique involved, and vaccinators rarely attempted to revaccinate a person who did not get a take. Smallpox continued in some communities, despite reports of high vaccination coverage. Finally, case reporting was both delayed and incomplete.

The vast gap between the goal of 100 percent vaccination and the low take rates, plus primary vaccination rates as low as 50 percent, was discouraging, but the value of independent assessment had been demonstrated. This study's pursuit of the truth set the tone for the frequent admonishment to smallpox workers in the 1973 campaign, borrowed from the American Management Association: "You get what you inspect, not what you expect."

In 1967, a year after the WHA passed the resolution to establish a funded global smallpox eradication program, a joint Government of India and WHO assessment team was organized. Four states were selected for evaluation: Maharashtra, which had a high incidence of smallpox; Uttar Pradesh and Punjab, which had intermediate incidence; and Tamil Nadu, with a low reported incidence. Within each state, districts and villages were selected at random for investigation.

The results were depressingly similar to those from the earlier evaluations. The number of reported vaccinations was high—494 million in the five years from 1962 to 1966—but only 70 million of these were primary vaccinations. And over 83,000 cases of smallpox were reported in 1967—the highest number in a decade and the second highest number of reported cases since 1951. The report also noted that India accounted for 65 percent of all reported smallpox cases in the world. If this was not enough bad news, the surveys in these four states indicated that despite all of the attention given to smallpox in recent decades and improvements in reporting, only one case in ten was coming to the attention of the authorities. Thus approximately 830,000 cases of smallpox had actually occurred in India in 1967.[28]

While the usual recommendations were repeated—better coverage and more attention to vaccinating children—several recommendations

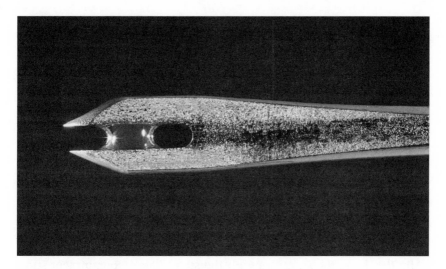

Figure 9. The bifurcated needle: inexpensive, dependable, and easily used. CDC/ James Gathany

were of historic significance. One was that every outbreak must be investigated by a medical officer to establish the diagnosis, trace the source, institute containment actions, and notify other districts as required. Another was a call to replace the rotary lancet with a newer, more efficient, and less expensive vaccination tool, the bifurcated needle, which had just been successfully tested in field trials.

Developed by Benjamin Rubin at Wyeth Pharmaceuticals, the bifurcated needle was incredibly simple and had several advantages over the jet injector.[29] The bifurcated needle was a simple steel rod with two tongs that when dipped into vaccine held the right amount for one vaccination. The vaccinator simply held the needle at right angles to the skin and pushed. The length of the tongs prevented going too far into the skin. Studies showed that removing visible dirt from the vaccination site was sufficient; cleaning the skin with alcohol, soap, or acetone was unnecessary. The field trials showed that the technique was easy to teach, provided take rates of 98 percent or higher, and required only about 20 percent of the vaccine used with multiple pressure techniques.

The needles were also inexpensive, costing about a half-cent each, and they could be reused, after sterilization, dozens and even hundreds of times. Supplies were lightweight and could be taken easily from door to door, and vaccinators could, under good conditions, do up to five hundred vaccinations in a day. A single individual vaccinator could not do as many vaccinations as with a Ped-O-Jet, but the ease of training and the ability to deploy large numbers of vaccinators using the bifurcated needle more than made up for that deficit.[30]

The various evaluations, especially the one by the National Institute of Communicable Diseases, had an impact. The Government of India was determined to demonstrate its interest in eliminating smallpox and was especially stung by the report that it harbored two-thirds of the world's smallpox cases.

By this time, the successes with the surveillance/containment strategy in West and Central Africa were well known, and D. A. Henderson, at the WHO office in Geneva, kept pushing India to incorporate it into its smallpox programs. In an August 4, 1967, letter to the WHO regional director in New Delhi, Henderson wrote, "Additionally, emphasis must, of course, be placed on active surveillance and containment measures."[31] This directive was passed on in the Central Government's letter to the various states regarding the fourth five-year plan, which began in April 1969: "It is vitally important for the success of the eradication program that right from the beginning emphasis must be placed on surveillance. This consists of smallpox case detection, immediate reporting, epidemiological investigation and the prompt institution of containment measures. Cross-notification of smallpox cases should invariably be practiced in all suspected import or export of cases. A system should be developed whereby all categories of medical and health staff are required to participate in the prompt notification of smallpox cases."[32]

Through the years of that plan, at a time when the exchange rate was about Rs. 7 to the dollar, the Central Government steadily increased its support to the states from Rs. 7.72 million in 1969–70 to Rs. 28.55 million in 1973–74. The number of vaccinators was increased in both urban and rural areas to about one vaccinator per twenty-five thousand persons, with a supervisor for every four vaccinators. In each district, one paramedical assistant was provided for every seven blocks—a block including about one hundred thousand people; there were over five thousand blocks in all of India. Each of the 386 districts had a mobile squad of five vaccinators that could be sent to any area as required. The Government of India assisted states in reaching this staffing level, in addition to providing other primary health workers who would be available in districts and blocks. This was an incredible army of people, approaching thirty-five thousand in number, assembled for smallpox alone. It would have taken astonishing foresight to have seen that within a couple of years, this would be only the core of a much larger army concentrating on smallpox.

The international community also stepped up assistance. WHO provided four long-term special epidemiologists and an average of three short-term consultants for two months each year, in addition to the staff working at the Southeast Asia Regional Office (SEARO) in New Delhi. The epidemiologists were assigned to the states with high incidences of smallpox.

Finally, in 1972, the reporting system was streamlined. The earlier system was based on the date of disease onset, which makes sense for the epidemiologist trying to determine rates of transmission, seasonal changes, and delays in reporting, but leads to endless and complicated record keeping. All reporting was changed to the week of report, no matter how long the delay in reporting. It was a breath of fresh air.

In addition, a weekly reporting network was organized. The Primary Health Center (PHC, usually the same as a block) was responsible for collecting reports from the entire block, subcenters, and local staff, as well as sending a weekly epidemiologic report to the district health officer. The district health officer then consolidated these reports into a single district report that was sent to the Directorate General of Health Services. The states reported by district to the central government and the WHO smallpox workers. If no smallpox cases had been detected, the PHCs, districts, and states were expected to send a "nil" report anyway, to differentiate "no report" from "zero cases reported." Experience had shown that people who forget to report a disease often have no qualms of conscience; they see it as a simple mistake. However, they will not falsify the record by reporting no cases if they actually saw cases. This requirement improved the accuracy of reports.

By 1973, the USSR had donated 1 billion doses of freeze-dried vaccine. WHO and the United Nations Children's Fund (UNICEF) provided equipment for India to manufacture its own freeze-dried vaccine in four facilities, located at Patwadangar in Uttar Pradesh, Hyderabad in Andhra Pradesh, Belgaum in Karnataka, and Guindy in Tamil Nadu. One of the great success stories of this campaign is the fact that by 1973, India was producing all of its own freeze-dried vaccine. The four producers settled on a protocol that used buffalo calves, stringent aseptic measures, and a standard seed virus. They also developed their own techniques for freeze-drying. Even dependence on imported ampules ended when the facility in Patwadangar developed an indigenous ampule that could be sealed by machines. Indigenously produced peptone was used as the stabilizer, and the final product met WHO standards for purity, potency, and stability. The national reference vaccine was shown to be stable even two months after storage at room temperature.

Everything was falling into place: government commitment, increased national and international resources, increased vaccination staff, sufficient vaccine of good quality, an easy system for vaccinating using bifurcated needles, a timely reporting system, and cross-notification of cases between districts to provide a national approach. However, smallpox was still not disappearing. Reported cases increased by over 25 percent between 1970 and 1971, and then increased by over 50 percent from 1971 to 1972. It was a confusing time as efforts escalated and yet smallpox did not diminish. Some people began to wonder if smallpox was indeed divinely inspired.

In fact, India was on the threshold of discovering the truth about just how pervasive smallpox was, which was the first step in loosening the virus's historic grip on the country. A new surveillance approach would provide that truth.

SEVEN Unwarranted Optimism

By the end of the summer of 1973, my family and I had settled into a new life in New Delhi. Everything was an adventure at first—money, school, shopping, the making of friends, and we adjusted once more to the heat and humidity of the tropics. I began work with the WHO smallpox team headed by Dr. Nicole Grasset at the SEARO office, which was in charge of the smallpox program for all of South and Southeast Asia. There was never any question, however, that our main focus was on India. We worked closely with health officials in the Central Government's Ministry of Health in New Delhi. As decisions were made, various people from both offices moved in and out of what became an informal leadership team for India's smallpox eradication effort.

India had been rapidly moving toward using the surveillance/ containment strategy in its smallpox program, and SEARO's assignment was to help the country implement this method nationally and especially in the endemic states. As the program unfolded, the populous

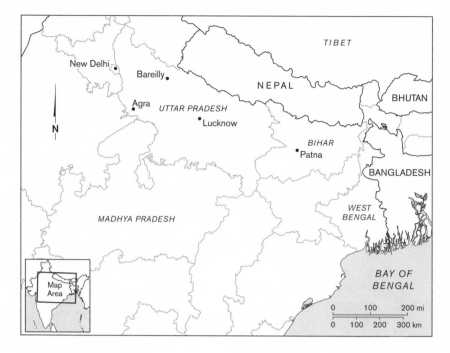

Map 2. Northern India

state of Uttar Pradesh, directly east of New Delhi, and its neighboring state to the southeast, Bihar, emerged as having the most challenging smallpox conditions. Dr. Grasset asked me to concentrate my efforts on those states while advising on the programs elsewhere in the country. The other two smallpox-endemic states were Madhya Pradesh and West Bengal. Containing the virus in these states would go far toward eradicating it in the country as a whole.

TRAINING THE TEAMS

By October, the smallpox leadership team had organized the first searches in Uttar Pradesh, Bihar, and West Bengal. That matter-of-fact statement disguises an incredible amount of work accomplished by a huge army of people. From the beginning, extremes dominated the work in India. First was the heat, which for much of the year was stifling, a fact of life that had to be ignored to be endured. A second factor was the size of the population, which was well beyond the experience of any U.S. public health worker. In 1973, Uttar Pradesh had 88 million people in fifty-four districts; Bihar had 56 million in seventeen districts (later thirty-one, as the state reorganized during the campaign). A third was the population density. While related of course to population numbers, the crowding factor presented challenges of its own. The areas of highest smallpox transmission in India were also the areas of highest population density. In many districts, the goal of 80 percent vaccination coverage through mass vaccination risked leaving more people susceptible to smallpox in every square mile than would be found in the United States if no one was vaccinated.[1]

What exactly was a search? The specifics varied by state and time, but searches were usually conducted monthly in the endemic states. For the six days of the typical search, a vast team comprising every health worker available (except those designated for the containment work that would follow) was mobilized to help find cases of smallpox. At the end of the six days, the daily hires were released, people working in other programs such as malaria and family planning went back to their regular responsibilities, and most of the other smallpox searchers were deployed to augment the containment teams.

A state meeting was scheduled to take place about two weeks after the search. This allowed enough time to assemble and digest the reports and prepare for the meeting, where refinements would be made for the next search, scheduled for one or two weeks later. The ministry and WHO staff worked quickly to develop guidelines as well as the forms required to implement those guidelines. A high level of trust and efficiency soon developed among the individuals involved.

Planning a search required developing a search protocol to be followed in an entire state, including estimates of personnel requirements at each level. Health officers could then arrange to borrow as many workers as possible from other programs and hire day laborers to make up the difference. We also developed model operational guides for both smallpox-endemic states and non-endemic areas.

Training courses were required at every organizational level. A training session was held in New Delhi for the health officers who would be overseeing smallpox operations in each state. This was followed by training sessions in each state for representatives of all the districts in the state. These district officers would then hold training sessions for each public health center (PHC, or block) in their district.

Each district had, on average, twenty such health centers with about one hundred thousand people in the catchment area for each center. For Uttar Pradesh and Bihar combined, there were 1,462 PHCs serving about 145 million people. Therefore, each district needed to train hundreds of people, and all of them needed to follow a similar protocol, keep records, report findings through a chain of command, and then assist in directing the containment workers as they were sent to control the outbreaks reported. The task of maintaining quality control throughout this hierarchy, and especially from the district training sessions to the almost 1,500 PHC training sessions, was overwhelming. Supervision followed the same pattern as the training—the district medical officers supervised quality in the PHCs, the state health officers supervised and evaluated the districts, and central government smallpox officers supervised the states. In the state of Uttar Pradesh alone, preparations for the first search required over 60 training sessions simply to get down to the district level, and an additional 930 training sessions at the district and PHC levels. I would sometimes think: this is a lot like the logistics of war.

The search teams were initially instructed to approach village leaders, mail carriers, schoolteachers, and students and to question people at tea shops or markets. In addition, they were to select two houses at random in the east, west, and central parts of the village to question the inhabitants. Each searcher had "recognition cards," small cards with the picture of a child with smallpox, to show potential informants. The look of disease is so distinctive that people knew immediately if they had encountered it recently.

Plans for containment efforts ran right alongside the preparations for the massive search effort. Containment teams were taught, forms developed, operating procedures agreed upon. There was, of course, no way of knowing how much smallpox the search teams would find.

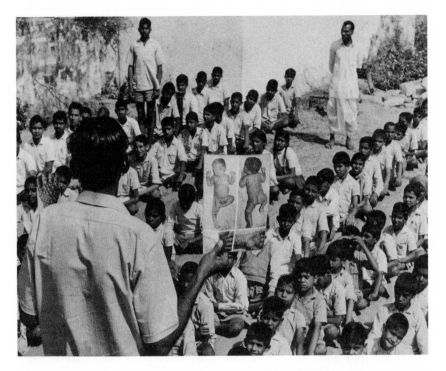

Figure 10. A search team member in India seeks information on smallpox using a recognition card

We based our containment plans on the current numbers of smallpox cases—and doubled it. According to the plan, containment teams in the PHCs would be the primary responders. District teams were ready to respond in case some PHCs had more outbreaks than their own containment teams could visit. State teams would assist where a district had more outbreaks than it could handle. We anticipated that containment teams would respond by vaccinating all susceptible members in households with smallpox as well as people in the twenty to thirty nearest households; this was included in the operational guide. A single-page instruction sheet was developed on vaccination techniques, use of the bifurcated needle, the preferred site of vaccination, and the sterilization of bifurcated needles after use (see figure 16).

In theory, since most smallpox transmission probably occurred within the home or in other intimate settings, vaccinating the susceptible people in households with smallpox cases would significantly reduce the probability of transmission.[2] The next most efficient vaccination activities would include other households in the neighborhood, family members in other neighborhoods, and other villagers who might have visited the sick person. Children who attended school during their first days of symptoms might also have transmitted the virus to others at school.

In general, different people were assigned to search operations and to containment operations. Asking the search workers who found smallpox to immediately begin containment operations might seem more efficient. It would avoid a delay in responding to an outbreak and avoid an extra trip to the village for the workers. However, experience in Africa had shown that this strategy was actually less efficient because there was a decided tendency to underreport cases if positive reports meant more work for the searcher.

Preparations required thousands of instruction sheets, training exercises, and reporting forms to be printed and distributed to thousands of searchers. But there was more. Although English is one of India's two national languages (the other is Hindi), not everyone reads or speaks English. So each form had to be translated into one or more of India's many regional languages. The training of supervisors and evaluators required additional forms and instruction sheets. This seemingly endless cycle of writing, translating, printing, training, and traveling might have seemed boring, but everyone involved was invigorated with the prospect of trying a new strategy under Indian conditions, despite the tremendous amount of work involved and the considerable risks.

The Central Government, states, districts, and PHCs were all agreeing to disengage health workers from other important activities for six days a month. They were also agreeing to a dramatic change in the way India approached smallpox. There was no guarantee that a strategy that had worked in Africa could work in an area with such high population densities. The variety of cultural differences in India, and the patterns of travel, with many people on trains and roads at any one time, also posed challenges. Not the smallest of the risks was the insertion of foreigners into village situations. Foreign workers were regarded with suspicion, and the smallpox team worried constantly that some kind of misunderstanding might embarrass or even jeopardize the entire operation.

Looking through the records from those times decades later, I am struck by how often I was optimistic while simultaneously having no idea what I was talking about. For example, because the first three searches were scheduled during the low-transmission months, I had written in the operational guide, "During October and November, the number of outbreaks will probably be small"—words that would come to haunt me. Just as naïve were the guideline words suggesting that every outbreak should be immediately reported by messenger without waiting until the end of the six-day search period. It would have been impossible, even in India, to enlist the thousands of messengers required to fulfill that mandate.

THE FIRST SEARCH

All of the planning culminated in an army of thousands of workers in Uttar Pradesh and Bihar fanning out for a reality test. The first search for Uttar Pradesh and Bihar was scheduled for October 15–20, 1973. Other states chose other start dates depending on local events. The prime minister, Indira Gandhi, put out a proclamation urging people to support the effort. The minister of health for Bihar opened the organizing meeting for the first search with words that evoked the image of a general sending troops into battle:

> We are meeting today to launch the final phase of smallpox eradication in Bihar State. The world is now depending on our success in this venture and I request your best efforts to see that we do not fail. . . .
> Chief emphasis during the next three months will be placed on two activities. The first activity is to find all cases of smallpox. . . . The second activity involves control of each outbreak with the help of health staff at block and district levels and by special State teams and WHO teams. Since this strategy has worked well in 27 countries over the past 6 years I fully endorse applying the strategy in Bihar State and

propose the highest priority be directed towards smallpox until it has
disappeared.

I must caution you that the key ingredient of the campaign will not
be words or money or vaccine but will instead be the dedication with
which each of you approaches this historical campaign.

I wish you a good meeting, a good campaign and I look forward to
the day when we all can enjoy a smallpox-free Bihar State.[3]

On the morning of October 15, workers departed from the headquarters of 1,462 PHCs. Each PHC searched twenty to twenty-five villages a
day for six days, from Monday through Saturday. By the end of the week,
over two hundred thousand villages had been visited in the two states,
and the PHCs started to tally the results. Within days the results began
to flow into the seventy-one districts. After district totals were compiled,
the results were forwarded to the states. It was like a river drainage
basin with hundreds of thousands of small streams forming creeks of
information, the creeks forming rivers; the delta they flowed into was
the assembly of all of this information for these two states.

In Uttar Pradesh, a state meeting of field personnel was scheduled for
November 5. The New Delhi staff began to worry that the meeting might
be chaotic if we received the district reports from this first search at the
meeting itself. The caliber of revisions in methodology for the second
search might be compromised for lack of time to properly consider the
results. It was decided that during the week immediately following the
search, I would canvas as many districts in Uttar Pradesh as possible
in five days. Then we would review what I found and use this limited
sample as the basis for preliminary recommendations for the second
search.

The program provided me with an Indian-made jeep and a driver.
The driver spoke no English, and I soon discovered he was unable to
read road signs in either English or Hindi. The Indian roads were a continuing challenge: a mixture of people walking, people on bicycles, rick-
shaws, scooters at times carrying four or five people, motorcycles, farm
vehicles, bullock carts, large trucks, buses, cattle, camels, goats, chickens,
varying widths of roadway, potholes, disregard for road rules—in short,
chaos. This would have been trying even if we were not also contending

with heat, dust, and diesel fumes, a cacophony of noise, and constant changes in speed. (We were stopped at one roadside safety check where the only test was whether the horn worked.)

At each district headquarters we would get detailed instructions for the driver on how to get to the next district. Yet getting lost several times a day became the constant. The variable was the length of time that elapsed before we knew we were lost. In scenes that reminded me of a Laurel and Hardy movie, we would stop, I would ask for directions in English, and the person would advise the driver on how to proceed in Hindi. For five days and nights, I gathered material and reviewed the findings as we drove. We stopped for meals, but to save time we did not bother to stop to find sleeping facilities. Rather, one of us would try to sleep while the other drove. Arriving at a new district headquarters, we would sleep in the jeep until the offices opened. After I had met with the district officers, we would be off to the next district.

It was in the middle of one of these night drives, with no moonlight, when my height presented a problem that could have been fatal. I was driving, my knees pressed against the dashboard, and one knee nudged the light switch, turning out the headlights; in the darkness, I was not immediately aware of why the lights had gone out. There was a moment of panic at forty-plus miles per hour, and then I realized what had happened and turned the lights back on. Despite the narrowness of the two-lane paved road, which barely allowed two trucks to pass each other, we were still on it! I have no idea how we escaped hitting the trees that the British had so thoughtfully planted long ago, which lined each side of the road.

The results of our trip were at first intriguing, then sobering, and finally scary. The search teams were finding far more smallpox cases than we had anticipated. We had based some of our expectations and many of our predictions on the passive reporting of the previous weeks. The number of new cases reported each week, for Uttar Pradesh and Bihar combined, had been in the hundreds. Even if the true figure was twice that number, it would not exceed the capacity of the containment teams already trained.

It was not simply that outbreaks were larger than projected, or that areas with smallpox had more outbreaks than anticipated—both of which turned out to be true. The real surprise was that new outbreaks were being discovered in PHCs that did not even know they had smallpox and thought they had been free of the disease for some time. This was the flaw of the passive reporting system. Health workers at the PHCs were waiting for patients to come to them. But smallpox patients were not showing up at the health centers because they knew that the health service could not help them.

I worked on the figures as we traveled, trying to understand what they meant in terms of containment efforts but also wondering what we would tell searchers for the next month's search. Would there be more surprises, or had this six-day search provided us with the truth? The last day of the five-day circuit required a stop in the city of Agra to meet with district health officers to discuss search results. We did not even have the time to drive past the Taj Mahal.

As the driver began the drive back to New Delhi, I started to analyze the figures just received. We had not even made it out of town when fatigue overtook the driver and he ran into a light pole, creasing the radiator and making the vehicle inoperable. While we were shaken by the incident, seat belts prevented serious injury. With a focus on the work at hand that is difficult to comprehend thirty years later, the driver and I shrugged off the incident and immediately shifted to solving the problem. Within twenty minutes, I had secured a district car and driver, and continued on my own to New Delhi. The driver stayed behind to fill out the accident report and arrange for repairs on the vehicle.

After I reached New Delhi, I began to feel the effects of the five-day trip. I developed herpes zoster (shingles) in a nerve pattern that involved the right side of my face below my eye. Within days I proceeded to Lucknow, the capital of Uttar Pradesh, to attend the first state meeting. The zoster lesion was weepy and hurt a great deal. At the Lucknow meeting, I was glad to encounter Dr. Gordon Meiklejohn, chairman of the Department of Medicine at the University of Colorado and one of the world's experts on herpes viruses. How could I have been so fortunate that a world-class herpes expert had volunteered as a short-term smallpox worker in India? He examined me and gave me reassurance. Months later he told me that he had nearly sent me back to the States because he feared the virus might extend into my eye.

The sample drawn from the five-day trip had been a warning. But at the meeting, as the reports from the fifty-four districts came in, we realized that we were in fact facing a disaster. In September, via the existing reporting system, Uttar Pradesh had reported 437 cases of smallpox. Now, just one month later, searchers had found 5,989 new cases. To put this in perspective: in only two of the previous ten years had Uttar Pradesh reported more than 7,000 cases in an entire year. Now, to the surprise and regret of the smallpox workers, it was found that 87 percent of the reporting districts—including 1,483 villages and 42 municipalities—had been harboring smallpox.

At Bihar's state meeting, the search team reported 3,826 new cases. However, the figures were incomplete because of inadequate staffing, so it was not even clear how many of Bihar's 587 PHCs had smallpox cases. Even with incomplete reporting, the search revealed that 477 of the 50,000 villages canvassed in Bihar, and 13 of its 103 municipalities, had smallpox cases. Smallpox was reported in sixteen of Bihar's seventeen districts.

The first search had identified almost ten thousand new cases in only two states. In the two states combined, 90 percent of all districts had smallpox and two thousand villages were involved, some with multiple outbreaks. In addition, 10 to 26 percent of all urban areas had smallpox. At a time when we anticipated a low point in numbers, we found smallpox everywhere.

On the one hand, we were euphoric at having pulled off something this unprecedented. Everyone praised the searchers for finding new cases, and they in turn were pleased with their results. In Uttar Pradesh in particular, health workers seeking smallpox had managed to get into almost 99 percent of the state's 140,000 villages and do at least a cursory search for smallpox in the short span of six days. That was no small feat.

On the other hand, the numbers signaled a daunting amount of work to respond to the search findings. We were in well over our heads. Indeed, the program did not have enough containment teams to travel to every new outbreak, even if they did no vaccinations.

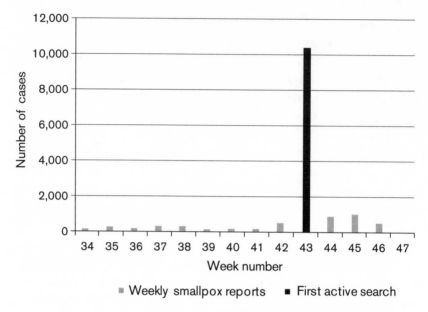

Figure 11. Smallpox reports from weeks 34 to 47 in Uttar Pradesh and Bihar, India, 1973

Some smallpox workers at the state and federal levels argued that we should cancel the next month's search and concentrate on containment, since it made no sense to find more cases if we could not control them. Some even suggested that we stop this form of surveillance entirely, as it made the medical system look inadequate for not reporting the cases earlier. However, the situation was overwhelming precisely because this was the best surveillance effort India had ever undertaken. The search had revealed what actually existed, not what we hoped existed. Keeping the truth in front of us would force us to respond appropriately. Our response should be to improve containment, not dumb down surveillance. The lesson for combating smallpox, and indeed for all public health programs, is that you can't form an effective response until you know the truth.

The central smallpox team decided to put at least a cursory effort into containment after the first search. We did our best to increase the number of containment teams, and they were told to concentrate only on the families with smallpox and the adjacent houses, rather than trying to vaccinate twenty to thirty nearby households, as the guidelines specified.

At the same time we tried to draw lessons from the first search in order to improve the next one, which was to take place just a week after the meeting. For example, searchers had noticed that schoolchildren were some of the best informants. They knew what was happening in their own neighborhoods and were not as reticent as their parents. There was also a hint of competition in the classroom to be the person giving the information. One new directive was to ask children if they knew anyone who had smallpox.

Everyone avoided discussing the possibility that the problem was so immense that it might be unmanageable. Instead, the focus was on how to address the barriers to eradication.

Many years later, Harlan Cleveland, a respected American political scientist, diplomat, educator, and author, observed that global health workers were fueled by "unwarranted optimism." That phrase well describes this band of smallpox workers as they took on the biggest public health challenge they had ever faced. It wasn't a case of putting a spin on the reality of the situation in order to fool others. If anything, we were fooling ourselves—though not totally. After the first search, the SEARO office in New Delhi sent a request to the WHO office in Geneva to provide up to sixty additional special epidemiologists. Needless to say, when the Geneva officials received the request, they were shocked.

THE SECOND AND THIRD SEARCHES

Armed with new information and with the experience of the first search fresh in mind, the search teams in Uttar Pradesh and Bihar moved out across the landscape for the second search on November 12. The results showed that the search teams had already improved their skills. Reporting was more complete. In Uttar Pradesh, again almost 99 percent of the villages were searched, but the searches were more effective.

During the three weeks between searches, another 800 new cases had been reported through the passive reporting system that was already in place. Hopefully this number constituted most of the backlog, and the numbers were now close to accurate. In fact, the second search revealed another 1,711 new cases in Uttar Pradesh. The situation was even worse in Bihar, where 2,459 new cases were found. Some of the new cases were within outbreaks found the month before. Others were in new villages but were quickly traced to outbreaks uncovered the previous month that had been poorly contained. However, far too many of the new cases had no connection to recent outbreaks. This meant that these cases had either been missed the month before or had resulted from outbreaks that had been missed.

The program was still far short of the ability to respond adequately to the level of smallpox being found. Resources for containment were stretched to the limit, and health personnel, supervisors, and trainers were not available at the levels required. Should the containment teams stay at an outbreak until all susceptible persons had been vaccinated, even if it meant not responding to all outbreaks? Or was their time best spent going to all outbreaks but doing an inadequate job at each? Either decision was an unprofessional, slap-dash approach to a very serious situation.

The compromise, unfortunately, was to do both, that is, to do an inadequate job at every outbreak visited and not reach some outbreaks at all. The smallpox team's "unwarranted optimism" allowed us to hope that vaccinating even a small number of people who were at highest risk would impact disease transmission, just as small increases in humidity and reductions in wind velocity can dramatically improve the efficiency of firefighting efforts. On this point, our optimism was trumped by reality.

One of the first changes introduced after the initial search was to shift the focus of attention from smallpox cases to smallpox outbreaks. This shift was made in Uttar Pradesh more quickly than in Bihar. The practical implications for control were the same whether a village had one, two, or twenty cases of smallpox. Both the number of cases and the number of outbreaks continued to be collected and reported, because WHO was using number of cases as the global metric. However, the number of outbreaks was the real indicator of the containment work required in each state, district, PHC, village, and municipality. It remained one of the program's most meaningful metrics.

At the end of the second search, using the new reporting system, Uttar Pradesh recorded 514 outbreaks that were pending, that is, requiring all of the attention and work of containment. The third search, held December 10–15, revealed 1,148 new cases and a total of 306 new outbreaks in Uttar Pradesh. New cases and new outbreaks do not correlate directly; for instance, the 1,148 cases were among the new outbreaks but also included cases reported from previous outbreaks that week in various stages of containment. In general, the median per outbreak was 5 cases.

The monthly improvements in searches were making it clear that Bihar had by far the biggest problem with smallpox in India, even though its population was only one-third that of neighboring Uttar Pradesh. During the third search, Bihar workers found 406 new outbreaks, with 2,619 new cases. Furthermore, whereas the first search had revealed smallpox in sixteen of Bihar's seventeen districts, it was now clear that all seventeen districts were infected. The first search had missed smallpox in an entire district, with a population numbering in the millions. As of the third search, over 25 percent of all PHCs in the state had cases of smallpox, and in the district of Bhagalpur, 80 percent of the PHCs were infected. It was almost impossible to travel anyplace in Bhagalpur without encountering smallpox.

REFLECTIONS AFTER THE THIRD SEARCH

In the final three months of 1973, the team learned a lot about what needed to be done to scale up the surveillance/containment strategy so that it would be adequate to confront the reality of smallpox in India. Each month saw changes in how the searches were conducted, the addition of new and complementary search techniques, and better approaches to record keeping and containment. The year ended with a system of smallpox detection that seemed to work. Certainly it far surpassed the effectiveness of the old passive system.

By the end of the year, most outbreaks were being visited by a containment team, even if the visit was weeks after the report and inadequate in actual containment. The containment team visits also supported the surveillance effort, since people are more likely to provide information when they have seen that it brings a response.

The light being shed on India's smallpox situation was gradually increasing in intensity. We were coming to know what was true, and this was inspiring everyone at all levels, from the central team to the PHCs. Knowing the truth has a way of inspiring belief and optimism that the job can be done, even when the job is overwhelming. The continuing optimism helped us to maintain the level of work.

In effect, the surveillance/containment strategy was a learning program, and experiences were regularly analyzed so we could figure out what would actually work in India. For example, it took time to find the most efficient ways of eliciting information. The fact that the residents had seen someone with smallpox did not necessarily mean they would pass on that information. They could be reluctant to share what they knew for many reasons. The solution was to have searchers, if they saw cases of smallpox, record on the reporting form for the village where the person lived and how he or she could be found.

Some experiments showed us what didn't work. For example, hoping for a shortcut, the central government/WHO team tried using presearch reports to indicate where searchers would most likely find new cases, but they proved useless. Districts that reported more than 20 cases of smallpox in the five weeks before the search averaged 133 new cases during the search. In districts averaging fewer than 10 cases during those five weeks, 139 new cases were found during the search. Even districts that reported no cases for the preceding five weeks averaged 67 new cases. The search itself, then, was the first reliable indicator of where smallpox would be found. This meant that searches had to be extended to every district in the state. There weren't many shortcuts.

By the end of the year it was also abundantly clear that even with barely trained search teams, the new system was more efficient than

India's old passive reporting system. It doesn't take a great smallpox tracker to find more cases than someone who is not out looking. The weak link in the program was the inadequately trained and insufficient number of containment teams; it would take them months to dig their way out of the morass of outbreaks discovered by the search teams, and this hurt morale. Again, we were saved by an unexpected finding: even poor containment teams were able to slow smallpox transmission.

Perhaps most significant, the smallpox workers were learning and improving every month, while the smallpox virus, for all of its evolutionary success, could not respond with the same agility. It continued in the way of its ancestors, unaware that its strategy for survival, adequate for millennia, would soon no longer suffice.

In the other two states where smallpox was endemic, West Bengal and Madhya Pradesh, monthly searches were also conducted through the fall of 1973. In West Bengal, all sixteen districts reported smallpox. Importations were frequent from neighboring Bihar and Bangladesh, but surprisingly, only 74 new cases were detected during the first search, for a total of 143 outbreaks listed at the end of the search. At the end of December 1973, the state listed 124 active outbreaks. While most countries of the world would have declared an emergency with a single outbreak of smallpox, much less 124, West Bengal was nevertheless a manageable problem compared to Uttar Pradesh and Bihar.

During the first search in Madhya Pradesh, 192 new outbreaks were detected, 53 during the second search, and 49 in the third search. These outbreaks were reported so early in their development that two-thirds of them had three cases or fewer, and 40 percent consisted of a single case. Madhya Pradesh's outbreaks were also limited geographically: only three districts had more than five new outbreaks. This was another manageable problem compared to Uttar Pradesh and Bihar.

Ten other states reported smallpox during these early months of the campaign, but all of them combined reported fewer than two hundred cases each week. Therefore, in most of India, while the problem had to be taken seriously, the containment of outbreaks was well within the state health systems' capacity and required little in the way of resources from the Central Government or other countries.

By the end of the third month, then, the smallpox program in India had developed its main themes. First, to eliminate smallpox it is necessary to know the truth; therefore, surveillance was the highest priority, followed by containment. Second, both surveillance and containment needed constant improvement. Third, we were all in this together. A unique group of Indian and international workers was clearly functioning as a team.

EIGHT

A Gorgeous Coalition

Mahatma Gandhi once said: "Interdependence is and ought to be as much the ideal of man as self-sufficiency. Man is a social being." Whatever people set out to accomplish requires teamwork. Every team does not work together efficiently or effectively. The vast team that came together to eradicate smallpox in India achieved both.

KEY MEMBERS OF INDIA'S TEAM

By 1973, smallpox eradication had become such a priority in India that the best possible people in India's Ministry of Health were assigned to it. Such a statement may be fashionable, even diplomatic; in this case, it was also true. In addition, over six hundred high-level supervisory personnel were eventually deployed from the central and state governments as well as from medical colleges, hospitals, and even private industry. These were in addition to the tens of thousands involved at the state, district, and PHC levels actually doing the searches, vaccinations, and outbreak control. Some states, such as Andhra Pradesh, contributed over fifty supervisors to the task. The Maulana Azad Medical College in Delhi provided ninety staff members. At a crucial point, Tata Industries, in an incredible contribution from the private sector, provided over a hundred high-level supervisors and actually managed smallpox eradication in a large geographic area of Bihar. With time, I came to realize that it would have been impossible to find a better team, even with a global search.

India's top health official, Dr. Karan Singh, took an active interest in the program. His background was impressive. He was regent of Jammu and Kashmir at the age of eighteen and later governor of that state, and was India's tourism minister before becoming minister of health and family planning in 1973. He set up periodic briefings with the smallpox team, asking useful questions and displaying both a quick mind and great managerial abilities. He especially liked the idea of setting monthly objectives for every state as well as conducting the monthly meetings in smallpox-endemic states, which provided a rapid exchange of information and obligated program directors at central and state levels to be involved in the field.

Dr. M. I. D. Sharma, head of the National Institute of Communicable Diseases (NICD), became in time the wise person to whom everyone turned. He had worked for many years in India's malaria program, had a comprehensive understanding of the Indian medical services, and was highly respected in the Indian states. He had participated in many international meetings. He never had to raise his voice to command people's attention. A large man, he might have been intimidating, but he was so kind and gentle that some likened him to a large teddy bear. He was known for his integrity, and when he requested people to do things, they complied without hesitation—not out of fear, but because they trusted him.

Although Dr. Sharma exuded calmness in the most difficult situations, there were telltale signs when his patience was reaching its limit. One such sign was that he began to rub his head. This would soon be followed by a very deliberate statement to end whatever argument was disturbing him. He would then, with good manners, move the meeting to a conclusion. On one occasion at a meeting of both Indian and foreign workers, an epidemiologist from outside of India was forcefully condemning the work of some of the medical workers. He became more animated as he continued, and Dr. Sharma began to rub his head. He did not interrupt the speaker but waited until he had finished and then said quietly, "Let me remind you that this is our country." The meeting continued on a very different tone.

Dr. Sharma enjoyed laughing, even at himself. Once as he and I waited to cross the street at an intersection in Patna, Bihar, he said, "Let me tell you what happened to me once at this very intersection." While he was waiting to cross the street, he told me, a rickshaw approached carrying a woman of such beauty that he could not stop staring at her. He was shaken from his spell when the woman greeted him by name. Seeing his confusion, she identified herself as a classmate from medical school. Flattered, he asked how she had recognized him after so many years. She replied, "I recognized your nose."

Dr. Sharma received bad news with equanimity and immediately set to solving the problem, and he received good news with the phrase, "God is good!" In one person was combined scientific acumen, managerial savvy, and a rare sensitivity.

Dr. P. Diesh, India's additional director-general of health services, was at first an enigma to me. On our initial meeting, I was disturbed by the way he treated a female colleague and his subordinates in the Ministry of Health. I was sure I would never warm up to him, only to find him a close friend within the year. It took me months to realize that his gruffness was his way of communicating his authority, which he exercised not to aggrandize himself, but to make the system work. He became a powerful force in guiding the Indian bureaucracy to embrace smallpox eradication. People would fall over themselves to comply when he barked out his orders. It was a surprise, then, to hear him express his fears and doubts as well as his concern for those carrying out the orders he gave. He wanted to be sure they had good working conditions and the support of their supervisors.

Diesh was dependable, had high standards, and could get things done. He also had the courage to take truth to power, including correcting the minister of health when he thought the minister was wrong. He knew everyone in government, enjoyed impressing an outsider with that network, and could make a call to solve almost any problem. Given his position, he did not have to get involved personally in the smallpox eradication effort, but he took a personal interest in the program anyway, attending state meetings and making field visits—indications of both his managerial style and the importance the government was giving to the program.

His pleasure on receiving a good cigar was so great that I would at times offer him a cigar while saying, "I have a great idea." We soon were joking that the idea did not even need to be a good one for him to agree; all I needed was a good cigar. Twenty years later, as we reminisced over lunch in New Delhi, he said that he had given up tobacco and alcohol and returned to being a vegetarian. He told me that he could never believe how shameless I had been in plying him with cigars. I told him that I could never believe how easy it had been. We reminisced about the smallpox program and our many discussions on field trips. Diesh said it was such a high point in his life that if I returned to India, he would come out of retirement and we could tackle another health problem.

Another key member of the Indian smallpox team was Dr. Mahendra Dutta, one of the most valued assistants to Dr. Sharma at NICD. His work in public health was part of a family legacy. His father had received a Rockefeller Foundation grant to study public health in the 1930s and later became the health commissioner for New Delhi. After the completion of the smallpox eradication effort, Mahendra Dutta in turn became the health commissioner for New Delhi. Mahendra's son, Dr. Umesh Parasher, followed the family tradition and became a brilliant public health worker at the CDC in Atlanta.

Dutta was the epitome of deliberateness and common sense in both speech and action, and was totally unafraid of fieldwork and all of its discomforts. He was given the job of providing central government supervision for the smallpox program in Bihar state. During the intensified smallpox campaign, he traveled almost continuously, attending meetings, making field visits, analyzing data, and solving problems. Early in the program, he discovered that a leader of Bihar's state staff was diverting smallpox resources for his personal use. This man was listing vaccinators who did not actually appear at work. For the use of their names on the employment rolls, they would receive their pay, despite no work, and split the money with him. Once this issue came to Dutta's attention, he was relentless in seeing to it that the man was replaced, despite the difficulties of removing an entrenched government leader.

Dr. Mahendra Singh was in a class by himself. As deputy assistant director-general of health services (smallpox), he had the longest institutional memory regarding smallpox of anyone in the ministry. He was the sole medical officer in smallpox at the central level from 1966 until 1972, with an impossible job: trying to hold back the relentless tide of smallpox virtually single-handedly. Before the government got serious about smallpox, Singh was working tirelessly to both fight smallpox and convince everyone from the central government level to the field that more resources were needed to do the job. Report after report showed his tenacity in promoting smallpox eradication before others accepted it as possible. For years he continued his uphill battle to tame smallpox; the obstacles were many, but he was never discouraged. He was the gold standard for a dedicated field-worker.

Two of the youngest members of India's central-level smallpox team were Drs. C.K. Rao and R.N. Basu. Rao, from NICD, was assigned to Uttar Pradesh as a central government supervisor because of his solid dependability and competence, and after his smallpox career he continued to be highly productive in the Indian medical service. Basu, who as assistant director-general of health services (smallpox) answered directly to Diesh, traveled widely to inspect field operations and continued to work in India and for WHO for three decades after the last smallpox case, using his experience and expertise for immunizations in general. Dr. R.R. Arora, a top epidemiologist at NICD, became a dependable and tenacious member of the team.

THE SEARO TEAM

I was fortunate to work alongside some exceptional people in SEARO. Dr. Nicole Grasset's dedication was unsurpassed. The distinction between days, nights, and weekends seemed to be irrelevant to her as she charged ahead with flair and courage. If Indian government officials at one level did not provide a positive response, she would go to the next higher level, and if that didn't work, she would go to the prime minister. Comfortable in any situation, and as charming as she was beautiful, she could endure the most difficult field conditions and also make sophisticated presentations at a conference or to the minister of health. Outcomes were her measure of a person, and she would give anyone a chance to contribute. She never lost her focus.

Grasset was also tough. During the drive back to our respective homes following an evening meeting with Diesh, I asked why she had been so subdued and seemed to hold back in promoting an idea she was developing. She responded that she was passing a kidney stone and was experiencing renal colic. This involves one of the most severe pains known and regularly incapacitates people, but it didn't stop her. Neither did her dedication to work keep her from appreciating the beauty around her. One time when we were waiting for a meeting to begin, she called my attention to the scene outside the seventh-floor hotel conference room in Lucknow. Outside, a light fog had covered the city, and streetlights shone like jewels through the fog. She said, "That is the way expatriate children see India, as a land of diamonds without the illness and pain and poverty."

At the conclusion of the smallpox eradication effort, she drove from New Delhi back to Paris, through Pakistan, Afghanistan, and Iran. This was not an uncommon trip for two or more people to make; rarely did a single individual do it alone.

Dr. Zdeno Jezek, a physician originally from Czechoslovakia, was accustomed to working under difficult conditions and had spent some years in Mongolia. While smallpox eradication attracted many type-A personalities, Jezek was the type-A gold standard. He seemed to have a well-thought-out speech always formulated in his head, ready for any occasion. Once when a speaker merely mentioned his name, Jezek jumped to his feet and began a rapid-fire delivery of a speech. Full of enthusiasm for the work at hand, he led others to do things by example. If he was ever discouraged, we did not see it. Even before we finally had smallpox on the run, he continued day after day as if each day would be the turning point.

Dr. Larry Brilliant, an American physician, had come to the Indian subcontinent to find truth, not smallpox. He learned the language, studied the country, and studied himself. When his guru told him it was now time to share his gifts by working to eradicate smallpox, he went to SEARO looking for a job, and Grasset was clever enough to provide one. Brilliant brought to the work a sincere interest in India as well as the desire to make his life count and to use his training to promote health. He could inspire local workers to see that it was not just a job, but a way to do good that would ripple through the coming generations. That is what karma is about.[1]

AN ALLIANCE AT THE CORE

It was more than good people that made the program succeed. An alliance formed between the Central Government and WHO that transcended all expectations. The reason for this alliance is complex. It may have formed because we traveled together, spending time with one another on trains and in jeeps, sharing lodgings, meals, and conversation. The rapport that develops through such experiences cannot be replicated by meetings in an office. We shared the moments of discouragement and the moments when things went right. The alliance formed not only because we developed respect for each other, but because we ended up trusting each other.

The shared travel was not a calculated choice. It happened almost by accident. In the beginning of the program, the WHO staff would travel between New Delhi and the state capitals by plane. One day Nicole Grasset and I were sitting at a table in the Patna airport, waiting for the daily flight from Patna to New Delhi. I said, "Nicole, does anything at the next table strike you as odd?" She looked at the two men, obviously pilots, seated at that table and answered, "No." I responded, "We know there is only one flight to New Delhi. Therefore the pilot and copilot at the next table must be for our flight. And they are drinking beer!"

I resolved to stop flying. It was easier, more dependable, and apparently safer to take overnight trains between New Delhi and either

Lucknow or Patna for monthly meetings. In addition, I could use the time on the train both before and after the meetings to analyze data. As it turned out, the real value was that the Indian smallpox leadership— Drs. Diesh, Sharma, and Dutta—also traveled on these trains, which provided the opportunity to talk in a casual setting. Soon we could predict each others' responses, and we found that we were thinking alike. As the insider-outsider barriers evaporated, an openness developed that helped to buffer both sides from problems within their own administrative structures. These train discussions, sometimes continuing in the sleeping compartments before we drifted off to sleep, helped us to work out the most difficult situations. When the Indian government could not provide an adequate per diem for the necessary field visits of Indian workers in the states, we faced that problem together and found a way for WHO to provide the funds. When all of the WHO resources had to go into surveillance and containment and WHO/Geneva could not provide additional money for evaluation, we were able to develop an approach with the Government of India.

The alliance formed to the point where it was unnecessary to develop guidelines on how we would operate. We reached decisions together. Our allegiance put us in a position of facing the world of problems united, rather than wasting effort in competing with each other. If anything, our competitive impulses were directed to competition with the virus. One of the lessons learned about collaboration is that the best ones begin with a clear vision of the last mile, rather than developing around a common interest and then laboring to define desired outcomes and identify a strategy. Smallpox eradication in India exemplified this. It also demonstrated a second important law for successful collaborations: the need to suppress egos and seek satisfaction in a shared outcome rather than holding individual power or protecting turf.

One distinction between the majority of collaborations and the ones that turn out to be especially productive is that the effective groups literally form a new substance. In chemistry, a mixture retains all the characteristics of the ingredients. A compound, on the other hand, forms a new substance with new characteristics, for example, when oxygen and hydrogen become water. The best alliances cannot be described simply by identifying the members. The sum is something different; it is a new compound. The objective becomes a shared objective that supersedes competition for turf. The talents coalesce into something more powerful than simply the addition of talents.

At times the ministry's knowledge of its own country saved us from error. I argued early on for a reward system to help us find new cases of smallpox—an approach that had worked exceedingly well during the final phases of eradication in West and Central Africa. I thought we should implement such a system as soon as possible in India. The ministry people wanted to wait until we knew how much smallpox actually existed—we might not be able to afford rewards. They saved the program from disaster. With thousands of new cases found in the early searches, rewards at that time would have broken the bank.

As time went on, the alliance just grew stronger, which in turn attracted others to participate. Notable was the Swedish International Development Authority (SIDA), which provided resources at a critical time. SIDA's approach to assistance is one of the most enlightened among development agencies. Before committing SIDA to the smallpox effort, J. E. Tranneus, director of the New Delhi SIDA office, was careful to evaluate the program, the strategy, and the probability of success. Following his review, SIDA made a grant with no strings attached. We were free to use the money in any way we felt advisable. The only stipulation was that we had to provide adequate accounting for how it was used.

MANAGERS FROM THE CDC

From the very first days of the eradication program in Africa, it was obvious that fighting smallpox was not just a medical or scientific endeavor but was very much a matter of management. We did need science; we needed to make scientific observations to understand the epidemiology of smallpox, the role of population density, the impact of cultural practices, the influence of climate, the vulnerabilities of the virus, and the impact of public health tools and experiences. And, of course, we needed to document our clinical observations. However, the real problems were in implementing the strategy: developing routines, documenting the implementation of those routines, hiring the right people, supervising, motivating, and evaluating. We needed managers, administrators, and logistics experts—people who knew how to solve problems and how to get things done. The program would not fail for lack of scientists, but it could fail—even with the best strategy—if we didn't attract the very best managers.

When commodities or people were needed, my first thought was to ask David Sencer, the director of CDC. He always found creative ways to provide the needed people, equipment, and support. Over the smallpox years, he developed a reputation for delivering on every request made of him. CDC smallpox workers soon realized that if you asked him for something, you had better be able to use it, because you would be stuck with whatever you had requested.

It has been said that genius is seeing one's field as a whole. Sencer saw the public health world as a whole. He understood that a healthy United States required a healthy world and that involving domestic public health workers in the global smallpox eradication program directly benefited the health of Americans. Addressing smallpox internationally obviously reduced the risk of smallpox importations to the United States, reduced risks for Americans traveling, and reduced the costs incurred by vaccinating the entire U.S. population. But there were other benefits. Don Millar, by this time in charge of the domestic program for immunization, was instrumental in sending many CDC staff members to the Indian program. He once wrote me that if his three-month loan of people for the program in India did nothing to improve smallpox eradication, he still wanted me to request them because they returned to the United States as different people. Once they had faced the problems of a developing country, they were unwilling to put up with the simpler barriers they encountered in domestic program implementation. The investment of domestic resources therefore seemed absolutely logical, and Sencer was willing to send CDC workers to help in the global effort.

In November 1973, shortly after the first search, I sent a telegram to Sencer stating that we needed a capable manager to help us develop administrative systems to handle the overwhelming situation we were facing in India. It was indicative of Sencer's interest that I received a phone call within a few days from his deputy at the CDC, William Watson, who asked if he would be acceptable as that manager. Watson had served in the U.S. Army during World War II and then earned a degree in political science, after which he worked under Johannes Stuart, whose combined interests in political science and public health translated into his effort to stem the postwar rise in sexually transmitted diseases. Stuart recruited college graduates to trace the partners of people discovered to have a sexually transmissible disease and get them to treatment before they in turn could become transmitters. It was, of course, a form of surveillance and containment, and it required combining the attributes of a detective with the sensitivity of a psychiatrist and the insights of a political scientist, a person who could see connections. Stuart's cadre of highly educated activist public health workers eventually became the managerial backbone of CDC, and Bill Watson became a father figure for this group.

Upon his arrival in India, Watson went to work on setting up a management system, addressing matters such as adequate training programs, sufficient transportation for field-workers (including a way to have vehicles repaired out in the field), and distribution of funds to those who would need them—the practical issues big and small that can become serious obstacles if not thought through. He was succeeded by an equally outstanding manager, Stuart Kingma, who was the kind of person who not only built his own telescope but also ground the lens himself. Kingma was a superb and creative craftsman whose talents transferred easily to administration. A compulsive manager, Kingma left no possibility unstudied. Watson and Kingma were followed by a continuous flow of top-notch CDC managers assigned to the SEARO in New Delhi on three-month assignments.

Once Bill Watson had set up the basic management structure, it was a matter of adjusting as needed. We had a framework, and succeeding CDC managers were expert at maintaining the right balance between attending to the never-ending daily needs of the program and keeping their eye on the big picture. The smallpox eradication effort in India would not have worked without these individuals: they got funds to the teams in the field, secured supplies to print and distribute thousands of forms, developed joint approaches between WHO and the Indian government, assured oversight, moved workers in and out of the field (and the country), and responded to thousand of requests from field-workers needing more vaccine, more bifurcated needles, or approval to purchase supplies. It was never ending.

THE CAVALRY: THE SPECIAL EPIDEMIOLOGISTS

To deal with the overwhelming numbers of cases unearthed through surveillance, the program in India needed, alongside managerial expertise at the central level, additional public health professionals in the field. India's fourth five-year plan for eradicating smallpox, initiated in 1969, included a category of workers called "special epidemiologists." Some were trained epidemiologists who had worked on smallpox or other diseases. Others were medical specialists in internal medicine or infectious diseases. Some were public health managers, and some were simply people who had worked in public health programs in India or around the world and developed a reputation for solving problems; these were taught smallpox epidemiology as part of their orientation. As with the workers in the Africa program, many found their life's calling by working for a period of three months to several years as special smallpox epidemiologists.

They were the smallpox program cavalry—highly mobile, able to inspire, and in charge of particularly difficult geographic areas with high smallpox rates. Each special epidemiologist was provided with a vehicle, a driver, and a health worker—a paramedical assistant (PMA) who if necessary also acted as an interpreter—as well as funds to use for expenses, including hiring day laborers. Each three-person team was assigned to assist in a state, a collection of districts, or even a single district where smallpox transmission was especially high.

Initially these consultants were mainly Indians and included just a few outsiders. Some of the most knowledgeable and capable smallpox workers in the world were in India. A.R. Rao, who had published a textbook on smallpox, was without peer in the world.[2] But just as a prophet often lacks credibility in his or her own community, it proved difficult to make full use of India's own expertise, including that of Rao. In any case, even India did not have enough experts for the scale of the problem that we on the smallpox team now knew we were facing. Epidemiologists from other countries could augment India's resources, and the SEARO team had already requested WHO/Geneva to send sixty more. However, bringing more foreign experts to help with what India saw as its own smallpox problem was a sensitive matter for this newly independent country. My several attempts to discuss this delicate matter with Dr. Diesh were unsuccessful. He could easily see where the conversation was going and expertly changed the subject.

On one of those overnight train trips back to New Delhi, in late 1973 or the first weeks of 1974, the topic of bringing more epidemiologists from other countries came up again. In the hour just before we arrived back in New Delhi, we found agreement on the point that India clearly had the ability to eradicate smallpox without additional outside workers. However, if we were interested in speed—in India not being the last country to stop smallpox—then the credibility and energy of outside workers were assets not to be overlooked. This view of the situation so excited Diesh that he decided to go directly from the train station to see the minister of health, Karan Singh, to make the case.

Later in the day, I encountered a very subdued Dr. Diesh, the only time in two years that I saw him discouraged. Even before Diesh stated the reason for his visit, the minister asked why foreigners were working on smallpox in India when India itself had so many experts. Taken aback, Diesh said nothing about bringing in more outside people and simply reported on the monthly meeting we had just attended.

By now, however, Diesh and I were both convinced that bringing in more foreign expertise was the right thing to do, and we discussed ways of making the case. Within the week, Diesh had regained his footing and he revisited the minister to make his case. Yes, India could do this without any outside people or resources, but acquiring experts from around the world would increase the chance of an early success—perhaps even during the minister's time in office. And, drawing on the help of the international community would demonstrate the Indian government's commitment to eradicating this disease. Diesh succeeded in convincing the minister that making this a global effort rather than an Indian effort alone would greatly accelerate eradication. The minister agreed, but asked that a balanced approach be used, one that would increase the numbers of foreigners and Indians simultaneously.

Following the first search, SEARO had asked WHO/Geneva for sixty more special epidemiologists (this included both medical officers and managers doing fieldwork). Now that the Government of India had approved that estimate and requested the additional expertise, consultants joined the team through arrangements made by Geneva, as well as from various parts of India itself.

During the ensuing months, thirty countries provided 235 consultants, with the United States providing 100 of them. With its experience managing the first successful regional smallpox eradication effort in West and Central Africa, the CDC now became a source of both long-term and temporary personnel for the eradication effort in India. People with experience in the Africa program were eager to see the same techniques applied in a more difficult situation, and we in India needed them.

The new recruits, who were usually seconded for three months or more, came first to New Delhi for a three-day training course. For eighteen months, I had the privilege of being involved in the training of all international as well as Indian special epidemiologists. The training course included a review of smallpox, the technical aspects of search and containment (even as we were learning them), a case study, information on the procedures they were expected to follow, and details on forms, reporting, and the role of monthly meetings.

The three-day briefing also included practical things learned by other special epidemiologists. For example, drivers or other people could remove petrol from vehicles during the night, sometimes even during daytime stops, and sell it for extra revenue. Many workers had tried to solve this problem by having a lock made for the petrol tank. But a clever driver could have a key made, even if the epidemiologist retained the original key. And four or five liters of fuel could easily be removed without detection, especially since the driver had to travel an unknown distance, after dropping off the epidemiologist, to find his own quarters for the night. The solution was to provide accommodations for the driver wherever the epidemiologist spent the night, and to fill the tank at the end of the day and again first thing in the morning, with the driver paying for any petrol added in the morning that exceeded one liter. The driver himself thus had to secure the tank in a way that prevented others from removing fuel.

The teams of short-term epidemiologists brought a continuing supply of fresh energy and new eyes to the operations. The special epidemiologists turned out to be invaluable in providing the flexibility the program needed in responding to shifting conditions and the changes in tactics that followed each monthly meeting. It took good planning to be able to use three-month assignees effectively, especially when most of the foreign recruits were experiencing India for the first time. It required adaptation on their part, but the training program was of sufficient quality that the results were far better than many predicted.

Problems occasionally arose, especially involving the diplomacy of non-American foreigners being supervised by Americans, who in turn were working under the direction of the host country, India. Given the Cold War politics of the day, the situation was especially sensitive if the Indian officials were displeased by a Soviet worker. It was much easier, and less political, for an American to send another American home. Yet the problems were generally worked through to a successful conclusion.

In an attempt to get to know the trainees, I invited many of them to spend an evening at our home. As the program progressed, I sometimes invited foreign workers who had stopped in New Delhi on their way home after their time in the field. On average, Paula and I had guests two to four nights per week. Joseph, our cook, provided home-cooked meals of great variety and was remarkably flexible about adding more places for visitors at a moment's notice. We were generously rewarded by witnessing the breadth of experience and high motivation of people from around the world who had come to India to make a contribution. Our children loved the opportunity to engage with a kaleidoscope of new people, especially those from other countries.

Unexpectedly, these evenings also provided opportunities to assess the relative strengths of and make assignments for these temporary workers. On occasion, a new worker's affinity for alcohol would raise a red flag in my mind. Others expressed false bravado regarding their ability to solve any problem in the field. A few complained about their hotel room in New Delhi, raising immediate suspicion that they would not fare well in the field. Over the ensuing year, many short-term volunteers arrived, were trained, worked for three months, were observed over two or three monthly progress meetings, and were then debriefed. A few workers were unable to adapt and were retired early. Eventually, it became clear that certain qualities were indicators of how they would do. These observations improved the chances of placing the most likely to succeed workers in the most difficult situations. The experience also provided me with a lifelong approach to evaluating candidates for positions.

The first quality was absolute integrity. These short-term epidemiologists would be handling large sums of money to pay daily workers, hire vehicles, provide fuel, and the like. There was no efficient way to verify how many day laborers they had hired or how many vehicles they had rented, and resources were simply inadequate for inspecting travel vouchers and weekly expenditure forms in real time. In any case, a worker would likely be gone before any discrepancy was spotted, so it was important to start with people who did not require that type of supervision.

A second quality was cultural sensitivity. The workers would be operating in someone else's culture. How they treated coworkers, patients, village leaders, school teachers—in short, everybody—was crucial to their access to people, the type of information they collected, and the work climate they would leave behind.

A third quality was optimism. The assignees were about to enter a world of work that was stressful and a climate that could be debilitating, with few amenities to soften the day. They were about to experience poverty and, in a small way, share the pessimism that is daily reality for so many. A pessimist transplanted into such a situation was not likely to thrive and be productive. Even an optimist would feel despair at times. Many workers later described their three months in the Indian smallpox program as the most difficult work they had ever done and yet, to their own surprise, the most satisfying.

Fortunately, all three qualities are easily researched, even though they are not found in the usual résumé or recommendations by supervisors. It is not that hard for people to assemble an impressive résumé and list references who will give them a positive review. Coworkers and subordinates are rarely listed by an applicant, yet they are the ones who can say immediately whether the person under consideration is trustworthy, sensitive to others in the work environment, or optimistic.

One of the early special epidemiologists, Dr. Don Francis, became for me the prototype of the person needed to defeat smallpox. He later had a distinguished career in infectious diseases, designing and supervising the first human trials testing an AIDS vaccine in the United States and Thailand. Francis began his India work in Bareilly, Uttar Pradesh.

This was an area of many smallpox outbreaks. Don resided initially in living quarters belonging to the Clara Swain Hospital, which was a place of historical significance because it had been built by the first woman medical missionary to India. Clara Swain left the United States in 1869, arriving in Bareilly on a January morning in 1870 after an all-night trip in a horse-drawn wagon. She began seeing patients that same day. By the end of the year, she had established her credentials as a doctor and was also training local students. By 1874, she had established the Women's Hospital and Medical School, the first in Asia. She went to see the Nawab of Rampore, who had publicly said he would not allow a Christian missionary in his city. He was so charmed by this determined young woman that he gave her forty-two acres for the hospital and school. Now Don Francis was building on that legacy by using the medical complex as the base for his smallpox activities.

Because of his success at motivating large numbers of local health workers, he was eventually transferred to Lucknow to oversee, under the state medical officials, the smallpox operation for the entire state. Don, in turn, had the utmost praise for Rajendra Singh, the PMA who worked with him throughout his two years as a special epidemiologist:

When we first started together, [Rajendra Singh] was helpful, but rather quiet and respectful. He watched as I met with high-level officials to explain the new search and containment strategy. He watched as I went to the field to do my own search for cases of smallpox. And he watched as I went to villages with outbreaks to evaluate the vaccination or, if there wasn't any, to vaccinate myself.

Soon, whether it was controlling an outbreak in a village or meeting with a high-level official in the state capital in Lucknow, Singh knew what to do.

In the villages I learned to turn to Singh to ask him how to proceed, especially in villages where there was some resistance to vaccination or ill-founded concerns. Standing as straight as an arrow, he would gently raise his hand before a protesting villager and say, "Gul suno" (Listen to what I am saying). Then, with personal force and gentle words, he would convince even the most resistant person of the good of what we were doing.

He had equal insight into the complexities of higher levels of the Indian government. He would rapidly assess what was behind the problems we confronted. Then, quietly and in private, would let me know exactly what was standing in my way and whether or not there was a way to address it.

Especially during the first year, when the program was failing and smallpox was everywhere, I don't ever remember him getting impatient or complaining of the long hours or the days-on-end away from home. Indeed, he was always there to help. When the weather got unbearably hot or when the road was so dusty that we couldn't see where we were going, he would urge us onward.

After smallpox, Singh returned to Pilibhit and headed up the District's immunization program. In 2008, while working on polio eradication, I visited Pilibhit and was fortunate to find him. He retired from government service to run his farm and a private pharmaceutical supply business.[3]

THE MONTHLY MEETINGS

The foundation of quality improvement for the smallpox campaign was the monthly meeting held in every smallpox-endemic state. The monthly meetings brought workers from every district to the state capital—Patna for Bihar, and Lucknow for Uttar Pradesh. Attendees included between two and six people from SEARO and the Central Government, the state smallpox officer, state health and political leaders, district medical officers, special epidemiologists, urban health officers for the largest cities, and several people from blocks that were of special concern. There might be fifty to one hundred attendees, and while the meeting could be completed in a day, many workers came a day early or stayed an extra day to replenish supplies or discuss special concerns with state and central officers. The meetings were usually conducted in a government meeting hall with ceiling fans but no air conditioning. Coffee and tea breaks were part of the tradition, and lunch was served in an adjoining room.

The meetings were primarily to review the work of the previous month and choose tactics and goals for the next. They were also an opportunity to get real-time feedback from field-workers, pursue scientific inquiry, evaluate what was working and what was not, replenish funds and provide payment, and recharge the field-workers' enthusiasm, which could evaporate after a month of hard work in trying field conditions. No small part of the meetings was the opportunity for foreign workers to leave their isolation out in the field and blow off steam.

The meetings always reminded me of reports of similar gatherings in the United States a century and half earlier, when mountain men working throughout the Rocky Mountains as well as local Native Americans would once a year bring their beaver furs to an annual rendezvous, often on the Green River in Wyoming. Both groups would sell their furs, buy supplies such as traps, ammunition, and coffee, find out what was happening in the rest of the world, and after a week or so make their way back to the field.

There was always a period of chaotic human Brownian movement as people greeted each other before settling down for the proceedings. The meetings began with a review of what had happened around the world during the previous month in smallpox eradication, thus incorporating the field-workers, in close to real time, in the global effort. A competitive feeling developed, since despite the massive problems we were facing, everyone hoped India would not be the last country in the world with smallpox. The next meeting item, a review of results from other states of India, similarly fueled both hope and a spirit of competition that their state would not see the last case of smallpox in India. Best strategies used in other states were also reviewed.

The meeting then shifted to district reports. Besides reporting the basics—the number of outbreaks at the beginning of the month, the number of new ones found, and how many had been contained and thus taken off the books—field-workers shared innovations in everything from how to find previously unknown cases to how they improved the productivity of health workers and daily laborers. Innovation was encouraged; when we identified effective new practices, we moved quickly to replicate them. At the same time, we tried to reward field-workers for being transparent about unproductive strategies so they could be discarded. We also found out which areas were overwhelmed with outbreaks and needed more supplies or people.

The meetings ended with two practices. The first was to distill lessons learned from the collective experience of all districts plus other states and forge this into a statement of new tactics to be tried the following month. Second, targets were set for the month by district and for the state. Only once during the program were the monthly targets actually met in Uttar Pradesh and Bihar, but knowing what we hoped for under ideal conditions served to motivate every worker, from the field to the central level. The end of each meeting also involved decisions on personnel placement and deliberate efforts to encourage each other to keep working in the face of tremendous odds.

Often the meetings revealed that some special epidemiologists were so beaten down that they needed special attention or to be replaced. These were tough people; they did not say they were depressed or overwhelmed. Most workers, regardless of how tired they were, were excited about sharing what they had been doing, the tricks they had developed, and the small successes they had experienced; some, however, were so overwhelmed that they could not get excited even over their own presentations. Just as the smallpox virus left a trail, so did depression. They tended to express frustration with their staff or district supervisors, or even the strategy itself. They might express anger about expectations, living conditions, or paperwork. Occasionally their behavior reached a point where the Indian authorities would ask for their removal.

The first level of response was to plan a visit to their area of work. Some people simply needed someone to witness the situation, to offer ideas, or to commend their actions. Misery, like poverty, can be endured when shared. However, sometimes this was not sufficient; some needed a face-saving way of going home early. Usually, they welcomed the suggestion that they had worked too hard and needed relief. How could they communicate this to others? By saying they had become ill and had to return. They were relieved to be going home but had not been able to make that decision for themselves.

A recent book on the Indian campaign, authored by S. Bhattacharya and based on his review of WHO archives, comments on the high level of dissension in the smallpox program. Bhattacharya says that dissension is evident in the records within WHO, in conflicts between WHO and Indian workers, between smallpox and other health programs, between the central and state governments, and between health workers and non–health workers. He also describes the tendency of WHO to attempt imposing its will on India.[4]

While these comments contain some truth—there were strong differences of opinion within WHO, within the regional office, and within India's Central Government—dissent was far from being the driving force. In fact, the climate of the program in the field was quite the opposite—exhausting, frustrating, and confusing, certainly, but remarkably positive and collegial even during the most difficult periods.

Yes, the staff at WHO/Geneva had strong opinions on how things should be done, but any attempt to impose their views would have failed. On the other hand, no suggestion from Geneva or elsewhere was ever discarded untested simply because it came from outside the country. Indeed, international policies were tested every month in every state, and the monthly meetings provided feedback on what worked and did not work under local conditions. No suggestion from outside of the country was incorporated into the program without validating its appropriateness for India. The interchange between people on field visits, the collegiality of district and PHC meetings, and the fine-grained texture of the daily work were not necessarily captured in the archival record.[5] While dissent was real and even encouraged, the actual story is how the months of intense and continual involvement of workers at every level, as well as the constant stream of communications in real time to everyone involved, promoted a level of trust that overcame any disagreements.

In retrospect, I would say that rarely in my half century of global health experiences have I seen such an effective coalition of workers as the one that developed in India. The core of that coalition was the monthly meetings. Representatives from the Central Government, state ministries of health, and other key state agencies all heard the reports from the villages. The usual communication and relational limitations of a hierarchical system were avoided; everyone attended the meetings. The team concept extended from every village all the way to Geneva. In facing the common goal of stopping a deadly disease that itself had no regard for rank or status, the usual governmental barriers gave way to a new kind of order and openness.

Indeed, in my view, the single most important reason for the successful eradication of smallpox, after decades of ineffectual efforts in India, was the seamless coalition that developed between India's smallpox program leaders and the array of international participants involved. A coalition can have great energy yet yield poor outcomes because people stake out their own turf. This did not happen in the India smallpox eradication program. Rather, the key groups joined together—a chaotic collaboration in the beginning but increasingly disciplined, coordinated, and purposeful. Over time, dozens of other groups and special interests joined too, including UNICEF, bilateral agencies, health and nonhealth government agencies, nongovernmental organizations, church groups, laboratories both in India and abroad, corporations, and various volunteers. If a coalition can be described as beautiful, this group became absolutely gorgeous, a model for all future national and global health efforts. The result—the eradication of smallpox—was not an accident.

NINE Rising Numbers, Refining Strategy

The first four months of 1974 were whipsaw months. The seasonal low point for smallpox transmission had passed, and transmission was now naturally increasing. At the same time, the searches were becoming more efficient. While this efficiency was a source of great pride for the smallpox workers, especially the search teams, it also meant that the reported smallpox numbers rose dramatically.

Boring to some, the numbers were fascinating to the smallpox leadership team. Many evenings after dinner I would say good-bye to my family and head to the New Delhi station to catch the overnight train to Lucknow or Patna. The hours before sleep were spent talking with Diesh or Sharma or Dutta or preparing for the upcoming meeting. I was endlessly analyzing numbers, looking for clues regarding what was working and what needed to be changed. What should be emphasized at the state meeting or with the state health authorities? Where did we need to place more people or resources? I was always looking for something encouraging in the figures, both to bolster my hopes and to share with field-workers, who needed inspiration in the face of overwhelming problems.

Numbers consumed our days, became our compass, and guided our actions. American investors check throughout the day to see what the Dow is doing, and sports fans turn on the news each morning to find out the statistics for their favorite team. With the same fervor we scanned the reports of new, pending, and contained outbreaks from each major search as well as from the supplementary searches that gradually became standard in high-risk areas during the interim weeks. Even the passive reporting system, which had lost its credibility in light of what the searches revealed, provided some information.

New outbreaks gave us a measure of how much spread was still occurring. The number of pending outbreaks, which included all outbreaks with active cases as well as all outbreaks that had not yet completed four weeks without a new case, indicated how many workers were needed in a given area at any point in time. When an outbreak area went for four weeks without a new case of smallpox detected, it was declared "contained" and could be retired from the list of pending outbreaks.

Because an outbreak remained on the pending list for a month after the last case, that list emptied slowly. In fact, the list could show an increase even as the number of outbreaks was decreasing. Likewise, a report of an outbreak containment referred to work actually done a couple of months earlier. This overvaluation of pending outbreaks and delayed gratification of contained outbreaks was intentional, building in margins of security. It was much safer to make truth prove itself than to guess at the truth.

We tracked other metrics besides outbreaks. We looked at numbers of deaths and numbers of cases for some information, putting them into rates per hundred thousand people or per month, week, or even day. Sometimes, to integrate data from search weeks with data from other weeks, we would use moving averages, or the average number of new outbreaks or cases per week by including two weeks before and two weeks after the week being examined. All of these were attempts to see the problem from different perspectives, and sometimes the numbers didn't easily compare. What were the best measures? If I wanted to have a guess at the size of the problem in order to plan for work assignments, I would look at pending outbreaks. If I wanted to know whether we were gaining on the problem, I would compare new outbreaks and contained outbreaks for a geographic area. But if I wanted to see the full fury of what we were up against, nothing was as telling as new cases per day. That brought the problem down to the people and families hurt forever on that day. At the height of the conflagration, there were fifteen hundred new cases of smallpox a day in Bihar—one new case every minute.

While the hope had been to conduct a search every month, the scheduling didn't quite work out that way. The fourth search was conducted February 4 to 9, 1974, and the fifth search from March 18 to 23. The sixth search spanned the last few days of April into the first days of May. Through the twenty months of the intensified campaign, there were sometimes only three weeks between searches; once, there was a seven-week gap. Therefore, some of the numbers that follow will refer to specific searches while at times, for clarity, the reports will indicate the average number of outbreaks found or contained by week during a given period.

In Uttar Pradesh, the number of new outbreaks found in each search was between 330 and 750, and the number of pending outbreaks continued to increase, so that 1,759 pending outbreaks were on the rolls in April 1974. Previous experience had given us no way of comprehending the work involved in dealing with over 1,700 pending outbreaks in a single state. Yet the situation was even worse in Bihar state.

The third search, in December 1973, had revealed slightly over 2,600 new cases of smallpox in Bihar. During the fourth search, in February 1974, 5,821 new cases, involving all districts, were reported. In terms of new villages with smallpox, the number had increased by 1,170. (Large villages could have more than one outbreak, but for practical purposes, the number of new villages infected was nearly the same as the number of new outbreaks.)

By March the situation had worsened. The number of new outbreaks reported that month averaged more than 600 per week, increasing to 1,000 some weeks in Bihar alone. This was almost twice the number of outbreaks being contained, so the number of pending outbreaks continued to increase. During the week of the fifth search, the discovery of 2,345 new outbreaks in Bihar increased the total pending outbreaks to 3,683 after the contained outbreaks were removed from the list. Figure 12 shows the number of new and contained outbreaks in Bihar during the first four months of 1974, combining information from the monthly searches, secondary and tertiary surveillance systems, and the traditional passive reporting system, which continued to operate throughout the smallpox eradication program.

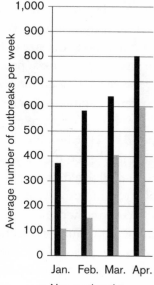

Figure 12. Average number of new and contained outbreaks per week, Bihar, India, January to April 1974

REFINING SURVEILLANCE

The numbers of cases and outbreaks climbed partly because surveillance kept improving. The monthly searches involved a frenzy of activity in districts and PHCs as health staff were diverted to the task of finding smallpox. Of course the remaining health workers were then left with increased workloads. Rarely are these workers acknowledged in accounts of the program, but they were absolutely key and should be counted as part of the vast army that comprised the smallpox warriors.

Every month saw innovations in search techniques. Early in the program the searchers began supplementing their earlier protocol by spending more time questioning children. Then the surveillance system moved from village searches—in which searchers would talk to key informants such as teachers, students, and village leaders—to going house to house in selected parts of the village. Eventually, searches developed to the point of going to every house.

The proficiency of the searchers grew month by month, both as a group and individually. Some searchers were more diligent than others, and switching searchers' assignments frequently resulted in detection of cases that had not been reported the previous month. That of course meant that those outbreaks had been free to expand.

The workers' objectives changed through the months, too. Early on, their objective might have been to correctly complete a form, but then they began to take pride in finding cases that they might have missed months earlier. Everyone was getting caught up in the challenge, and the concept of a team approach was infectious.

Surveillance also improved markedly as the program developed. At first, the surveillance approach was an extension of approaches used in Africa. Gradually, however, smallpox workers discovered how to do better surveillance, including how to identify both the population groups most likely to have smallpox and those most effective in hiding smallpox cases. The discoveries of individual workers, reported in monthly meetings, became the basis for improving surveillance overall. Secondary and then tertiary search techniques evolved, based on what was being missed by the six-day searches. The techniques were intended to be redundant, thereby increasing the likelihood of recognizing the presence of the virus. During the weeks between main searches, supplementary searches became standard in areas of high suspicion. There was a sense—later confirmed by the data—that the rate of identifying outbreaks and existing cases was increasing.

With experience it became possible to draw up guidelines for supplementary surveillance. Secondary search techniques involved sending teams to wherever crowds assembled—markets, fairs, religious ceremonies. Smallpox workers would go through the crowds with recognition cards, asking if anyone had seen a person with smallpox. The teams submitted positive reports to their supervisors, including the name of the person's village and whatever other information they could garner.

Tertiary searches were started for groups that were not integrated into the local community and thus not likely to be found in village searches. These included the Harijan communities (the "untouchables") and occupation groups such as road builders and kiln workers, who moved from place to place in search of work. Beggars were usually found at markets, in urban areas, or at railway stations; less often in villages.

The high degree of mobility in India presented another difficulty. Millions of people are on the trains at any one time, not to mention buses, trucks, and other vehicles. In addition to the usual reasons for travel, such as commerce and family visits, people would travel to fairs and religious meetings, which could draw more than twenty-five thousand visitors to a single site. The previous October, in Bihar alone, almost 8 million people had been expected to visit fairs. A single religious *mela* (festival) in Uttar Pradesh meant over 5 million visitors converging on a small geographic area. Special teams had to be deployed to search and vaccinate in these large congregations.

By January 1974, the searches that had become so useful in smallpox-endemic states were extended to the entire country. Searches of the non-endemic states were conducted every three months. To visit 100 million houses in six days' time, an army of workers had to be organized. The procedures that had become routine in the smallpox-endemic states now had to be replicated in the other states, districts, and PHCs. Tens of thousands of searchers, supervisors, and evaluators needed to be trained. It constituted one of the largest operations in public health history.

Every three months, the country obtained a snapshot of where the smallpox virus was hiding. When previously unknown cases were found in non-endemic areas, the teams had the capacity to respond quickly to avoid large outbreaks. The presence of cases in non-endemic states meant that the infection had been imported from an endemic state. The quarterly searches of the non-endemic states not only stopped spread from the endemic states but also indicated the origin of the cases, thus helping to pinpoint the problem areas in endemic states. This in turn put more pressure on those districts to protect both themselves and the rest of India.

IMPROVING CONTAINMENT

Improving containment was the key to responding to the soaring numbers. In early 1974, the huge gap between new outbreaks and contained outbreaks was beginning to narrow, but only slightly; yet knowledge of the field situation was improving at PHC, district, and state offices. By this time, the national operating instructions for the smallpox program called for a supervisor to actually visit each outbreak to evaluate the work of the containment team. That didn't happen right away, of course, because the ideal was always ahead of the actual. Also in early 1974, with a high degree of hope, containment teams were directed to return to the practice of vaccinating twenty households around each house with smallpox.

The number of outbreaks was so large that at first the containment teams were unable to respond adequately. They would vaccinate the affected households and immediately surrounding households but would then have to go to the next outbreak. Moreover, as the early months of 1974 progressed, the large number of outbreaks meant that even though there were more containment teams, they might not be able to visit the majority of outbreaks before the next search added even more outbreaks to the list. PHC and district medical officers were forced to prioritize outbreaks. With so many outbreaks, even basic record keeping, a minimum requirement, was a challenge.

Besides the rapid increase in outbreaks, the labor-intensive nature of outbreak containment and the difficulty of continuing to train more teams left the program constantly running behind in containment capacity. For each outbreak, an investigation was required to determine the origin of the outbreak and to notify the PHC that had exported the virus. Vaccinations, which eventually included census operations, had to be organized. The search had to be continued for weeks after the last case. Finally, the containment team had to close out the outbreak once the last patient had recovered. The amount of work, record keeping, and supervision for one outbreak was prodigious. Even after containment work had ceased, repeated visits were required for four to six weeks afterward to be certain no new cases had developed. These visits were followed by repeated visits from a supervisor to insure that protocols had been properly followed and the outbreak had been terminated.

The concept of a six-foot perimeter of no susceptible people around a smallpox patient proved to be a useful rule of thumb in stopping outbreaks. But, just as a forest fire can jump a firebreak under certain conditions, so the virus could occasionally jump this thin line. This was rare, however. Don Francis reported one of these unusual events. To commemorate the death of a young boy from smallpox, the family invited all of the village children of the same age to their home for a *kheer* (rice pudding) party. As the children were sitting on the front stoop of the house eating their *kheer*, the dead child's grandmother began cleaning the child's sickroom. She brought the bedding out to the front stoop and shook and beat the child's quilt next to where all the children were sitting. Ten days later, these un-immunized children all came down with smallpox.

It was soon discovered that people from outside the immediate family and even outside the neighborhood were expected to visit a person who was sick with smallpox, providing considerable opportunity for the virus to jump the six-foot perimeter. Forbidding visits was simply not enforceable; this rule, interpreted as an offense to the goddess of smallpox, simply drove the practice underground. The solution was to post watch guards at each patient's house with instructions to vaccinate every visitor. The watch guards were provided with journals and were expected to record the names of those they vaccinated, as well as their own food and bathroom breaks. Hiring, training, and deploying watch guards at each house was added to the work of the containment teams.

The numbers involved in just this small aspect of the program once again demonstrate the size of the containment actions. Posting two watch guards per house meant hiring and training ten new people for every outbreak (the average outbreak consisted of five cases). Five thousand pending outbreaks in Bihar meant a new workforce of fifty thousand people. Later in the year, the number of watch guards for each infected house was doubled to four to insure round-the-clock coverage. At the peak of the 1974 smallpox season, eight thousand pending outbreaks alone required between fifty and a hundred thousand watch guards.

Another problem was discovered when it was observed that family members or neighbors of vaccinated people were coming down with smallpox one incubation period later. They had been missed in the vaccination. Many were working in the fields, buying food or petrol, or engaging in other life activities. Some, however, were missed because they intentionally avoided vaccination, mistrusting anyone from the outside, especially government workers. Some were children who had been hidden by their parents.

Correcting this problem required an additional step. Before beginning vaccinations around an outbreak, the team took a census of surrounding households by asking an informant to list all the members of every household. In the evening, vaccinators or watch guards would concentrate on finding persons listed on the census form who had not yet been vaccinated. Explaining the rationale for vaccinations and enlisting the support of the infected village took a lot of time and effort.[1]

In fact, it was rare for anyone to refuse to be vaccinated. R. N. Basu writes, "In reality, resistance to vaccination in India remained a limited phenomenon without substantial influence on the program. . . . Generally speaking, less than 3% of the people . . . might be expected to refuse vaccination during a containment operation."[2] When someone did refuse, the risk was to the person not vaccinated, with little potential impact on eradication. If that person developed smallpox, he or she would be surrounded by vaccinated people and would be unlikely to easily transmit the virus.

THE VALUE OF EVALUATIONS

The value of knowing the truth applied not only to the incidence of smallpox but also to the eradication program itself. In training programs, in field visits, at monthly meetings, and in sessions with health leaders, this motto was emphasized: "You get what you inspect, not what you expect." Central and state program officers put this wisdom into practice by visiting district and PHC headquarters. Containment, as well as surveillance, improved when it was supervised and evaluated. Through the first half of 1974, it became increasingly common to enter a district health office and see maps and charts on the wall regarding the smallpox situation. By May, this practice was also common at PHCs.

As the year began, smallpox leaders had an array of informal ways to measure the quality of the program; these methods provided the building blocks for an increasingly formalized evaluation system. PHCs could compare how many villages a worker said he or she had searched with what the supervisors later found. Supervisors could see the wall markings left by searchers. The number of chicken pox cases the searchers reported, too, was indirect evidence of their efficiency in reporting smallpox. The number of new cases the containment teams found indicated the efficiency or inefficiency of a search, as did the amount of time between the onset of an outbreak's first case and the reporting of that outbreak. From the beginning, field experience provided data that were used to update the informal evaluation practices that were in place.

By the time smallpox peaked in April and May 1974, the program was able to send out evaluation teams. Building on the informal evaluation methods already in place, the teams used a marking system whereby containment teams were asked to make a mark on the door of each house they visited. The mark used was changed each month. An evaluation team later recorded the number of houses visited, and in a sample of houses, questioned the residents about what the searchers had asked as part of the search.

Throughout early 1974, evaluation was becoming more systematized, and by April, it was feasible to formalize the evaluation criteria. The key indicator chosen for evaluating the efficiency of surveillance was the time from the onset of the first case in an outbreak until the outbreak was reported. Typically, the first report of an outbreak was actually the second generation of cases. The first, or index, case was often a solitary case that the family was able to keep hidden. Since the second generation of cases appeared approximately fourteen days after the index case, and allowing for the time required to submit reports, we chose twenty-one days as the expected time from the onset of the index case to the report. The percentage of outbreaks reported within twenty-one days was therefore the key indicator of good surveillance in a district. The key indicator for adequate investigation efforts was set at 90 percent of outbreaks traced to a known outbreak. The measure determined for adequate containment was no new cases more than twenty-one days after discovery of the outbreak. These few indicators or "vital signs" made it possible to quickly spot deficiencies in searching, investigating, and containing outbreaks; such weaknesses could be related to particular PHCs, districts, or even individuals.

The WHO/New Delhi staff presented the evaluation plan to a visiting representative from WHO/Geneva. While WHO/Geneva was unfailing in its support of India's program and could be counted on to provide personnel, resources, vaccine, and political assistance, its resources were stretched so thin that it could not fund the proposed evaluation program. The Geneva representative left New Delhi the night of this decision. The next day, as a demoralized WHO/New Delhi group reviewed the program, they decided that the effort was so important that they would seek funds from elsewhere. The evaluation program was instituted and became an indispensable management tool and the driver for quality improvement during the last phase of the campaign.

A MOUNTAIN OF FORMS

Each new refinement in search and containment methods required training, new procedures for reporting, and new forms, which had to be distributed on an ongoing basis to thousands of PHCs and districts. India's vast bureaucracy, often maligned, was ideally suited for an operation of this scale. Indeed, once the power of the Indian bureaucracy was harnessed, there was no stopping the innovation and energy of the thousands who took on the challenge of defeating smallpox. Record-keeping forms may seem like humble soldiers in such an effort, but the form itself became the driver that led to the actions needed to achieve the desired outcomes. Creating effective forms requires you to picture the desired results, how to achieve those results, and how to report on them. Forms proliferated, and in a very real sense we can say, in retrospect, that smallpox was suffocated by a mountain of paper.

The following is a partial list of the forms that field-workers had to contend with:

Searching
    1. Workers' Schedule for Search Teams
    2. Workers' Schedule for Urban Areas
    3. Smallpox Market Search Book
Investigation
    1. Smallpox Outbreak Investigation and Containment Report (Form C)
Containment
    1. Smallpox Containment Field Book for Containment Teams
    2. Smallpox Outbreak Summary Booklet for Containment Teams
    3. Daily Work Diary for Watch Guards and Vaccinators
    4. Market Search Form
Reporting
    1. Urgent Notification of Smallpox Outbreak (postcard)
    2. Cross-Notification of Smallpox (postcard)
    3. Cross-Notification Book (outgoing—with four copies plus one retained form)
    4. Cross-Notification Book (incoming—with copies to be submitted when investigation complete)
    5. Weekly Epidemic Report Form (PHC to district)
    6. Hospital Weekly Epidemic Report
    7. Market Search Summary (PHC)
    8. Market Search Summary (district)
    9. Smallpox Weekly Epidemic Report (PHC to district)
    10. Supervisors' Report Form
    11. Weekly Checklist for Special Epidemiologists
    12. Weekly Report Form for Special Epidemiologists
    13. Weekly District Report of Pending Outbreaks
Evaluation
    1. Rural Search Assessment Form
    2. Urban Search Assessment Form
    3. Verification of Active Search Form
    4. District Search Summary Form
    5. State Search Summary Form
Protocol and Instruction Forms
    1. Search Protocol—Instructions for Searchers
    2. Case Finding Form for Searchers
    3. Guidelines for Market Searches

4. Search Assessment Protocol
5. Model Operational Guide for Endemic States (September–December 1973)
6. Operational Guide for Low-Incidence and Smallpox-Free States
7. Operational Guide for Endemic States (June–September 1974)
8. Guidelines for Eradication of Smallpox in Urban Areas
9. Operational Guide for Smallpox Eradication (January–March 1975)
10. Operation Smallpox Zero (after February 1975)

Record keeping was essential for understanding what was happening, and people filled out forms to the best of their ability—a legacy, no doubt, of the British system in India. Workers at all levels were encouraged to provide feedback. The information on the forms was incredibly useful in guiding the program. At the monthly meetings, field-workers would hear that information handed back to them in the form of refinements to the strategy.

POLITICAL MATTERS

During these first months of 1974, I traveled often. When not on trains to and from state meetings, I traveled by car or jeep to make field visits. Sometimes these trips went without a hitch, and sometimes the unexpected occurred. At the beginning of April 1974, I took our middle son, Michael, then age eight, on a field trip to the northern districts of Bihar. On our return, we crossed the Ganges River, a distance of over a half mile, by loading our jeep onto a small ferry. The ferry was so crowded that Michael and I sat on top of our jeep while our driver managed somehow in the crowd. In the middle of the river there was suddenly a great deal of excitement as the ferry began taking on water and people began to bail water with buckets and pans.

Assuming a calmness I did not feel, I told Michael that if the ferry did sink, we would take off our shoes and slip into the water. I reminded him that he was a good swimmer and that the two of us would easily make it to shore. The ferry made it to the south bank, and I thought the highlight of the day was behind us. It turned out I was wrong.

It happened to be April 8, the day that the famous Gandhian Socialist J. P. Narayan, at age seventy-two, led a silent procession in Patna to protest corruption in government and injustices such as hunger and rising prices—part of the student protest movement known as the Bihar Movement. As we drove toward Patna, we were unaware that because of the protest, the city was under a curfew.

At a stop sign, long before reaching Patna, our jeep was surrounded by students caught up in the protest. They began rocking the jeep back and forth with every indication that they planned to turn it over. Assuming a false bravado for the second time that day, I tried to reassure Michael, telling him this happened all the time, and I rolled down the window to talk to the students. They demanded money, a request that to me seemed totally foreign to the ideals of J. P. Narayan. They stopped rocking the vehicle as I got out to talk to them. I said I had money for them all and began distributing the smallpox recognition cards, telling them how much I would pay for each case of smallpox they identified. I continued talking, urging them to become part of the solution, to go into the villages and urban areas to find cases, to do this for India, and not only for India but for the reward I would give when they brought me cases. They stopped to look at the cards and hear what I was saying. That encouraged me to more forceful exhortations. Then they began to back away, possibly out of embarrassment or fear. As I spoke louder and with more fervor about what India was trying to do to rid the country of smallpox, I realized I had gained control. Gradually they retreated and finally disappeared.

We cautiously resumed our trip into Patna, passing burning trucks and buses tipped on their sides. Few other vehicles were on the road, and absolutely none as we entered Patna. The streets were empty, and an eerie silence filled this usually loud and crowded city. At the Republic Hotel, where I usually stayed while in Patna, a guard recognized our vehicle and opened the gate. The hotel management had taken up carpets and anything that might burn in case Molotov cocktails were thrown through the gate into the hotel entrance. Michael and I, along with our driver, remained there until the curfew was lifted several days later.

It was a politically tense period in India in other ways as well. It was the era of the Cold War and the Vietnam War, and the Indian government was somewhat suspicious of foreign workers, especially if their work took them into the villages. Indeed, in 1974, the newspapers in India began carrying stories that the malaria research work being conducted with U.S. resources and scientists in India was actually an effort by the CIA to develop biological warfare techniques. Once such stories start, they can become impossible to counter, even when they're groundless. The malaria studies were eventually suspended. About the same time, an American smallpox field-worker who was in New Delhi for a few days reported to me that during his meal at a restaurant the previous evening, a man sat down at his table and told him that the smallpox program would be next to receive that type of publicity. It never happened, but the warning served to keep us anxious.

As the early months of 1974 passed, more special epidemiologists joined the smallpox program until there were approximately one hundred special teams in the field. While they strengthened the regular health resources devoted to smallpox, and their effectiveness was a major factor in motivating the entire team and efficiently using field resources, there was also the constant worry that someone would embarrass or even jeopardize the entire program.

On one occasion, an American special epidemiologist who was working in the field and living in a military guesthouse sent me a commercial telegram. The military had asked him to seek other accommodations, and he was asking that we verify that he was not a CIA agent. It was a strange request but could not be ignored.

We at the WHO regional office would have been dismayed if the CIA had used any of our people and decided that we should be straightforward in asking if it did. I went to a friend at the U.S. Embassy and asked his advice. He asked another person—clearly, the head of CIA activities for the embassy—to join us. This person read the cable with concern and assured me that he knew nothing about this person.

He then asked, "How good is he?" I replied, "He is not that good." The embassy official said, "There are two hundred people eagerly waiting to read your reply. If you send him home, it will be interpreted as confirmation that he is a spy. He just bought himself some additional time with your program!" I sent the epidemiologist a bland reply discussing work and suggesting that he might want to move to a rest house.

Through the months, the political climate improved. So when I received a request one day in April to see the American ambassador, Daniel Patrick Moynihan, I assumed he wanted a status report on the smallpox program. I walked through the huge front door of the embassy, as always aware of the sudden transition from extreme heat to air-conditioning. I expected this to be fun, and was surprised to see the embassy physician, Dr. Ed Etzel, pacing the floor. He had been waiting for me. He grabbed my arm and said he had some advice: Moynihan thought one hundred times faster than anyone in the embassy, I should know that Moynihan was very angry with me, and I should not say a word. "Don't argue," he said, "because he will be merciless."

I entered the ambassador's office in a state of confusion—what was going on? The ambassador was standing at the side of his desk with an angry look on his face. With no niceties or greeting whatsoever, he said, "I have evidence in this folder that you are spreading smallpox rather than stopping it." Wow, I thought, what an opening gambit! He went on to explain that India's Communist Party was likely to announce that the United States had sent spies into India under the guise of working on smallpox. The office of the prime minister had asked for a meeting with him that afternoon for an explanation. I saw the presence of so many Americans in India as a scientific issue, but to him it was political, particularly given the number of Americans in the states of Bihar and Uttar Pradesh, near the Nepalese border. He was now in a difficult diplomatic position.

He continued heatedly at some length, without pause. I thought about Ed Etzel's advice, to keep silent, and realized that there was no alternative. Abruptly, he stopped and asked me again what I had been thinking and how in the world had I managed to get these people into Bihar near the border with Nepal without the embassy even knowing?

In fact, wanting to be cautious, I had made all of my requests to Dave Sencer for additional people from the CDC through embassy channels, rather than WHO channels, precisely so the embassy would know what was happening. For a fleeting moment, I considered telling him it was all spelled out in embassy cable traffic, but immediately thought better of it.

Instead, I began by describing how the world now had a chance for a historic first in eliminating smallpox, and the key to global success was India, and the key to success in India was Bihar. Bihar, I continued, had the highest rate of smallpox transmission recorded in the global program, with one thousand new cases a day in that single state. We had no choice but to put our attention in the place with the problem. Without enough epidemiologists, the effort would fail.

To my amazement, the ambassador made a complete about-face. He became truly interested and began asking questions. Finally, referring again to his impending meeting with Prime Minister Indira Gandhi, he asked, "What should I ask of her to speed up the program?" The Government of India—supportive of the program all along—subsequently deepened its support even more.

PREDICTING THE TURNING POINT

What I told the ambassador was no exaggeration. In the first four months of 1974, India reported more than sixty-seven thousand cases of smallpox, and over two thirds of them were in Bihar. When the numbers of outbreaks declined in Bihar, they would decline for the entire country.

A solid month before the official figures showed a decrease in pending outbreaks, smallpox officers knew eradication was possible and indeed only a matter of time. This became obvious by watching the increase in containment outcomes. In Bihar in January 1974, outbreaks were being taken off the pending rolls at the average rate of 107 per week. One month later, outbreaks were being retired at an average rate of 152 per week. This rate increased to averages of 403 per week by March and 596 outbreaks per week by the end of April.

Throughout this time, the number of new smallpox outbreaks increased dramatically, so the number of pending outbreaks continued to increase. But that, we knew, would not continue indefinitely. We were gaining.

New outbreaks measured new findings at that point in time and therefore reflected the current activity of the smallpox virus, while retired outbreaks indicated containment work that had been completed one to three months earlier—an outbreak had to be free of new cases for a month before it could be removed from the pending list. Thus there would always be a lag in the number of outbreaks removed from the books. In other words, the program was doing better on the ground than the numbers showed.

The searches had become more efficient; the average time from discovery of an outbreak until the last case in that outbreak was going down. Containment was growing more efficient, too. The average time from report of each outbreak to its closing out was also decreasing. Finally, the number of outbreaks removed from the pending list was increasing each week. By this time, no special insight was needed to envision the point at which the contained outbreaks would exceed new outbreaks. Once the pending outbreak list began to decline, it would do so at an accelerating rate. As the outbreak numbers declined, additional experienced troops could be assigned to contain each remaining outbreak, and containment efficiency would improve even more. The natural decline in the transmission rate once the rains arrived in June would assist the rapid clearing of larger and larger geographic areas.

The turning point was not far away. In early April, the number of contained outbreaks in Uttar Pradesh improved significantly, and in the space of a month it increased from approximately 100 per week to an average of over 250 per week. This was absolutely amazing progress. Because there was a four-week waiting period (of no transmission) before an outbreak was removed from the pending list, these numbers reflected program improvements going back to February. When we analyzed the trends, we could predict that the containment capacity in Uttar Pradesh would overtake the discovery of new outbreaks in May.

As for Bihar, the fact that over five hundred outbreaks were removed from the pending list each week in April was incredibly encouraging. In this area of high transmission rates—the virus was claiming over one thousand victims a day—we could project a decisive turnaround within four to six weeks. We knew we were close. The numbers told the story.

TEN Water on a Burning House

As the month of May began, a hot month in Bihar even by Indian standards, the number of smallpox outbreaks skyrocketed along with the temperature. The sixth search (April 29–May 4) had revealed 2,622 new outbreaks, the highest one-week total we would see. This brought the pending outbreak total to 4,921. The pending figure would have been even higher except that containment teams were by now so efficient that they were removing over 800 outbreaks per week from the pending list. More important, the number of new outbreaks was only slightly greater than the findings one search earlier, while the containment ability had doubled in two months. For the smallpox worker who knew what to look for, the expected tipping point was thus palpable at the beginning of May.

The fact that a single smallpox outbreak in a European country would be seen as an emergency, with untold resources deployed, provides some insight into the work required to address almost 5,000 outbreaks simultaneously in a single state. Workers in Bihar were stretched to the absolute limit. The situation had turned a corner on paper, but the physical demands continued. No one had ever experienced a public health operation of this magnitude before. (We did not know it yet, but through May, about 100 new outbreaks would occur per day, producing 1,000 new cases of smallpox per day.) One had to be an optimist with a feel for numbers to be ecstatic at the same time that Bihar had over 5,000 known smallpox outbreaks and had just reported over 11,600 new cases of smallpox in a single week.

I thought back to a conversation the previous fall with D. A. Henderson. WHO/Geneva was programming its computers for the 1974 global smallpox surveillance program, and Henderson asked me

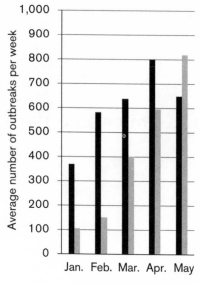

■ New outbreaks
▥ Contained outbreaks

Figure 13. Average number of new and contained outbreaks per week, Bihar, India, January to May 1974

to estimate the highest number of cases that we would have in any state of India during any week in 1974. Based on the reports in previous years, I replied: fewer than a thousand cases. Three digits in the column for cases per week per state would be sufficient. WHO, with an abundance of caution, decided to allow for a fourth digit. I saw no harm in adding a digit, so didn't protest. Now we were in the embarrassing position where even four digits was insufficient.

The number of pending outbreaks continued to rise, but we were euphoric because we could now see the breakthrough on the horizon. The gap was quickly narrowing between new outbreaks detected and outbreaks removed from the rolls. The psychological boost, which we were already feeling because of demonstrated success, would fuel even harder work on the part of everyone (figure 13).

A STRIKE, A BOMB, AND DOUBTS

Then, seemingly out of nowhere, a series of disasters came crashing down around our house of elation. On May 8, the railway workers went on strike. The program would have to hire trucks and drivers to move supplies. But that was not the real problem. India's railway system, a British legacy, was the backbone for transportation of goods and people, with a reputation for running on time. The railway was said to be the biggest housing project in India, with 1 percent of the country's population on trains at any one time. The workforce maintaining this system was enormous and had the largest, most powerful union in the country.

Other workers watched the railway union to see what was possible. The real implications of the railway strike became obvious when half of the vaccinators in Bihar went on strike to protest wages. The other half named a date later in the month when they would join their colleagues. The district medical officers followed suit, announcing a date in early June when they too would leave work. These decisions were made before the smallpox leadership team even knew there was a problem.

We quickly sorted through the options. There weren't many. Could we form our own health army by hiring thousands of daily laborers, using experienced workers as supervisors, and run the entire program under the auspices of district magistrates or other nonhealth segments of government? Meetings with district medical officers were not encouraging. Some were willing to help, but there was no way to re-create the size and expertise of the workforce being lost.

In utter frustration, and totally out of character, I lost my temper one day while talking to one district medical officer. I had asked if he would help me find the kinds of people I would need to hire when the strike occurred and develop plans to immediately switch to this alternate system when government workers left their jobs. With a condescending air, he said, "If there is no strike we would be wasting our time to develop an alternative plan. If, on the other hand, there is a strike I would have no interest in an alternative plan." I slammed my fist down on his desk with such force that books fell and dust rose. "What kind of a man are you, anyway?" I bellowed. The sudden fear in his eyes provided a small measure of gratification but no support, and I abandoned the effort with extreme frustration.

At least, I told myself, there is some comfort in knowing that things could not get worse. And then, from an entirely unexpected direction, the program was hit with a problem that could not have been anticipated by even the most diligent planners. On May 18, 1974, India detonated its first nuclear device. Reporters from around the world came to India to report on the event. When they ran out of new ways to report the same story, they looked for others. Suddenly, smallpox in Bihar became world news. Few of the dispatches bothered to explain that the program had greatly improved the accuracy of India's smallpox surveillance system or that the largest response the world had ever launched against smallpox was already under way.

In response to this negative publicity, India's legislators began asking very pointed questions about the quality of the health services, and some feared that India had become an international failure in the effort to eradicate smallpox. The international publicity and the attention of parliament now placed pressure on political leaders in the states.

Those supporting the new strategy were clearly on the defensive. The smallpox alliance was convinced that the vast number of cases, especially in Bihar, resulted from three things. First, it was the seasonal high period. Second, the efficiency of surveillance had finally cast a strong spotlight on what might have been happening every year—only no one knew it before. The truth of smallpox in Bihar was at last revealed. Third, there may well have been an unusually high number of cases that year, but there was no way to test this, since no year in the past had ever had such efficient surveillance. Convinced that containment procedures were rapidly gaining on the head start experienced by surveillance, we now wondered if we would get the opportunity to prove that assumption. We longed for the anonymity that had surrounded the smallpox program before the news crews arrived.

The response of the Indian smallpox team in the Ministry of Health was beyond compare. They were diverted daily from the task of smallpox eradication to answer endless inquiries. The minister of health, Karan Singh, was totally supportive. Some of the people in between were skeptics. Dr. J. B. Shrivastav, India's director-general of health services, was one such person. Though supportive publicly, he would privately say the smallpox effort was ill-conceived and doomed to fail, and he encouraged state ministers of health to abandon the approach. He had enough authority to be a problem.

In an interview with Myron L. Belkind, New Delhi bureau chief for the Associated Press, Shrivastav went public with his gloomy message. WHO workers had earlier told Belkind that despite the setbacks in Bihar, they had "all the necessary weapons: sufficient vaccine, adequate manpower and, most important, support from the Indian Government," and they were still envisioning an end to smallpox in India in 1975. When Belkind mentioned this optimistic projection during the Shrivastav interview, Shrivastav said that a more realistic goal would be 1979. "I wish it to be so but let us be realistic," Shrivastav said. "I'm an Indian and I know where I am situated."[1]

Shrivastav was of course not alone. Despite the success of the surveillance/containment strategy in other countries, many public health workers still held the view that CDC epidemiologist Henry Gelfand expressed in his May 1969 letter to Don Millar: surveillance/containment should be the primary strategy only "under certain circumstances"; otherwise it might be misinterpreted to "justify fruitless and inefficient epidemic chasing in India and Pakistan."[2] Now here we were "epidemic chasing" in India. If leading smallpox experts didn't think surveillance/containment could work as the primary strategy in India, no wonder there was doubt.

The field-workers, so weary with the heat, long hours, and difficult field conditions, were vulnerable to suggestions that their efforts were futile. Field people and supervisors alike were well aware of the "field paranoia" syndrome. I have been on both sides of that syndrome and know it is real. When things go wrong in the field and you have been working to the maximum, you conclude that the problems must be because headquarters is not providing appropriate support. And, there may be some truth to this claim. At the same time, however, one becomes blind to one's own errors in allocating time or resources. Field paranoia was often apparent at monthly meetings, where workers often expressed frustration with headquarters and made excuses for disappointing results.

One WHO special epidemiologist, originally from France but working in South America for the Pan American Health Organization, resigned with a sharp rebuke and stormed out of the country, saying his life was too valuable to waste on a strategy that couldn't work in Bihar, where he was assigned. Unaware of the expectation of a turning point in May or June, he wrote a long report in June stating that the current approach was failing and that his proposal for mass vaccination of the district, supported by many of the best smallpox experts in the world, had been rejected.[3]

In the midst of all of these problems, a great boost was given to the program in Bihar. Larry Brilliant was able to convince the heads of a giant corporation, Tata Industries, that the area around their plant in southern Bihar was one of the great problem areas of the state. Tata agreed to take on a large geographic sector, provide the medical and managerial staff, and work under the guidelines of the government's surveillance/containment program. Tata put some of its best staff on the project and stopped smallpox transmission in the area; by doing so, Tata freed up program personnel to be assigned elsewhere.

This amazing coalition of public and private sectors was a harbinger of the pharmaceutical philanthropy that would become commonplace a quarter century later. Merck contributed hundreds of millions of treatments of Mectizan for the control of onchocerciasis (a disease leading to blindness, the so-called river blindness) in Africa. Merck and GlaxoSmithKline contributed Mectizan and Albendazole to a global program for the control of lymphatic filariasis (a disease leading to swelling of legs and scrotum, also called elephantiasis). Pfizer provided Zithromax, an antibiotic, for the treatment of trachoma, a disease leading to blindness. Dupont enlisted one of its companies, Precision Fabrics, to provide filter cloth to strain drinking water for the prevention of guinea worm. GlaxoSmithKline and the Gates Foundation joined forces to develop a malaria vaccine. Merck and the Gates Foundation developed a demonstration program to show how twenty-first-century science could work in AIDS control in Botswana, reducing the HIV positivity rate of newborns from 35% to 3.5% in less than a decade.

BIHAR'S MINISTER OF HEALTH

The real price of the rising skepticism about the strategy didn't become obvious until Bihar's minister of health decided to halt the seven-month-old strategy in his state. Suddenly and unexpectedly, he simply withdrew his support. He had been supportive, but he was under intense political pressure from legislators and other political actors who had fallen prey to the power of the forces aligning themselves against the surveillance/containment strategy. The most politically expedient response was to return to the security of what India had done for over 170 years. Whether effective or not, the known was preferred over the unknown.

At first I thought he might be just testing us, but then it became clear he was serious. The weeks and months of hard work, the endless logistics and meetings, the hundreds of training programs and thousands of workers trained, the analysis and scheming, the constant jarring in a jeep, the sweaty nights under a mosquito net—they were about to become wasted effort. Did he have any idea that he was threatening to put the entire India program, indeed the entire global program, in jeopardy?

We would have to return to the basics and figure out a way to provide both the mass campaign required by the politicians and the things we knew would actually work. But I could not see at that moment a way to do that, certainly not with the resources available.

It wasn't the science that threatened to stop us. It wasn't even nature, per se. Rather, it was human nature: the human factors that involve strikes, job security, political concerns, turf. I remembered those words from graduate school: "When you tangle with culture, culture always wins." As hard as the daily work had been, this was the only time I was discouraged and uncertain about the outcome. I thought we had lost the battle.

Bihar's monthly smallpox meeting was scheduled for Monday, May 27, and the minister planned to announce his decision at the meeting. M. I. D. Sharma, Mahendra Dutta, and I met with the minister several times in his office and even at his home over the weekend. Over the months we had met with him often to brief him on progress, ask him to speak to the field-workers, and report the results of monthly meetings. But the meetings held that weekend reached an intensity not experienced in the past. Sharma and Dutta had the advantage of knowing the system, knowing how hard to press and when to back off. We begged the minister to give us another month to prove our strategy. A firm commitment to a date might well have swayed him, but we didn't have a precise date.

We pointed out that the strategy of mass vaccination had been unsuccessful in India for the better part of two centuries. He had tried the new strategy for a scant seven months. We were asking not for an extended period of time, but only for one more month. He in turn said that he understood our concerns but that the pressure was coming from everywhere, including his superiors in New Delhi, to revert to mass vaccination. We were unable to provide him with a single example in his entire state where a district was showing a decline in pending outbreaks. That is the point that separated us. We could see the inevitability of eradication as containment improved and new outbreaks increased but at a decreasing rate. The political pressure he was receiving required a decrease in the pending smallpox outbreaks in a few districts, not simply a promise that this would happen soon.

He kept returning to a single, worn argument: he had allowed us to pursue this new course, unproved in India, for seven months. During that time, no mass vaccinations had been done, and a backlog of unvaccinated children had been building. That backlog must now be addressed. He had no recourse now but to attend our monthly meeting on Monday and tell the assembled staff of his decision.

A YOUNG PHYSICIAN SPEAKS UP

With a profound sense of resignation, Sharma, Dutta, and I entered the meeting room on that hot, sticky Monday morning for the monthly routine. After seven months of intensive activities in Bihar, the staff in the field had increased, and eighty or ninety people crowded the room. Ceiling fans provided some air movement, but when the room temperature exceeds body temperature, even air movement doesn't yield much comfort. But these were field-workers, accustomed to hardship, and I watched with appreciation and some awe as they pressed on despite the heat.

I sat at the front table with Sharma, Dutta, and Achari (director of the smallpox eradication program for the state of Bihar), gazing at this roomful of very weary faces. The meeting opened with the usual greetings, followed by reviews of the world smallpox situation and the situation in the rest of India, a description of the programs in key states, and a summary of new and potentially useful ideas that had come out of other state meetings. Finally, we got to the review of the smallpox situation in Bihar, including the pressures that were on the minister of health to change the strategy. We shared the fact that the minister was preparing to ask us to change the strategy and return to mass vaccination. We also shared our discouragement in being unable to change his mind.

The minister suddenly appeared, flanked by an entourage, and strode to the front table. He was given the floor immediately, and he described the problem as he saw it. Bihar was now faced with fifty-seven hundred pending outbreaks involving every district of the state. He acknowledged that hundreds of outbreaks a week were being retired and that the heroic efforts of the workers had no precedent in public health history. But: the number of new outbreaks found each week was even higher, so the number of pending outbreaks continued to increase. It was clear to him that we were losing the battle. He saw no alternative but to revert to mass vaccination, and to do it quickly, before the backlog of unvaccinated children increased even more. At meeting's end, he declared, we would return to the strategy of mass vaccination in Bihar. We all knew this was coming, yet hearing the words actually uttered was shocking. Their impact began to sink in, and the room became very quiet.

One of the field-workers, a young Indian physician, raised his hand. He looked too young even to be a medical school graduate, and he was very thin, the epitome of a dedicated field-worker. He did not appear to have the needed gravitas for the moment, and I worried that a mistake was in the making. But the physician stood and, with great deference, addressed the minister. He was shaking as he described himself as just a poor village man. But, he said, when he was growing up, there were things you could depend on. For example, if a house is on fire in a village, no one wastes time putting water on the other houses, just in case the fire spreads. That is the mass vaccination strategy. Instead, as in the surveillance/containment strategy, they rush to pour water where it will do the most good—on the burning house.

Despite the heat of the day, a chill went up my spine as this man condensed all the work, discussions, discoveries, and massive human effort of the previous seven months into a few words and the indelible image of a house on fire.

The minister hesitated and stared at the group for some time. And then the unimaginable happened. He changed his mind on the spot. This man of public authority, who over the weekend had resisted the combined persuasive powers of Drs. Sharma, Dutta, and myself, this man who had entered the meeting room thirty minutes earlier with such presence and purpose, now seemed subdued, almost bewildered. He pointed out the great personal and political risk of his changing his mind. But he said, in a small voice, "I'll give you one more month."

Soon after, other things began to go right. The railway strike was settled that same day, and the other groups withdrew their strikes and strike threats. The monsoons arrived, and with them, a decrease in the transmission potential of smallpox.

The search conducted during the first week of June finally brought good news and the information we needed to influence politicians. The number of outbreaks decreased by over a third from a month earlier (2,622 to 1,678), the number of pending outbreaks did not increase (remaining at slightly more than 4,000), and even the intensity of cases per outbreak seemed to be declining as the number of cases found dropped from over 14,000 in the April/May search to about 7,500 in the June search. The change was sufficiently dramatic that we had no problem convincing the politicians—including Bihar's minister of health.

Anyone who has lived in India or Africa through the dry season knows the incredible surge of emotions and energy that accompanies the first rain. People dance in the villages and celebrate. This was the feeling of the smallpox workers when the smallpox problem in Bihar finally began to decline in June 1974.

ELEVEN Smallpox Zero

The arrival of a new vision just when people think they have worked to the maximum gives them new energy, allowing them to push beyond their previous limit. In early August 1974, the smallpox leadership team sent out to the field-workers in Bihar a graph showing the decrease in outbreaks reported in June. The same graph was distributed to all smallpox workers in India on August 26 as part of the seventh SEARO surveillance report. The whole team could see that their work had now paid off: we were on the downhill slope.

The turnaround in Uttar Pradesh happened at the same time as in Bihar, with 47 out of 54 districts infected in May and only 44 infected the next month. The number of new outbreaks peaked at 792 in June, one month later than expected, but then fell quickly: fewer than 50 new outbreaks were found four searches later.

The improvement in evaluation techniques initiated earlier in 1974 continued to pay off through the summer. Effective evaluation allowed

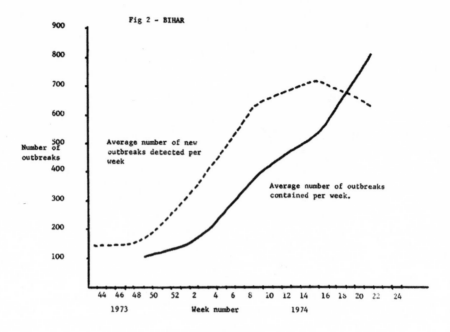

Figure 14. Graph distributed to field-workers showing the June 1974 turning point, when outbreaks in India began to decrease (see the dotted line)

us to redeploy resources with confidence that the highest priority needs were being addressed. At last we understood the enemy. Attention placed on measuring the efficacy of the program, the effectiveness of the various components, and the efficiency of operations allowed us to predict what the virus would do next. The intelligence gathered allowed us to outflank a virus that had the supreme confidence of thousands of years of finding new victims without a break in the chain of transmission.

Following a search, ten villages in a district were selected at random to determine whether searchers had visited. Attempts were also made to discover smallpox or chickenpox cases missed by the searchers. The time from onset of the first case until the outbreak was reported continued to decline. The percentage of outbreaks reported within twenty-one days of onset eventually reached 100 percent on a routine basis. A final test involved determining the source of the index case. Trails do grow cold, but most districts were reaching the target of tracing the origin of 90 percent of all outbreaks.

Containment evaluation also permitted comparison between districts. The standard was that no new cases should be found more than twenty-one days after discovery of the outbreak. For those going longer than twenty-one days, a detailed analysis was undertaken—in effect, an outbreak autopsy, which had been standard teaching fare in the forensic public health field so close to the heart of Alex Langmuir at CDC. Such detailed analysis made it possible to determine that incomplete or delayed containment actions were the primary reason for new and continuing outbreaks.

Assessment results were provided to states, districts, and PHCs by means of monthly reports. In addition, the results were discussed at every monthly state meeting and formed the basis for developing new tactics for the following month. By mid-1974, the results were dramatic, and resources were rapidly moved to correct the defects revealed by the evaluation techniques. In both June and July 1974, the number of outbreaks contained in Bihar exceeded the number of new outbreaks.

Several vectors converged, allowing the program to attack the last vestiges of the virus with increased force. As the number of pending outbreaks declined, staff were freed up from containment work. Improvements in containment, search techniques, and evaluation all helped to reduce the number of outbreaks and cases. As the caseload decreased, more attention could be given to each outbreak, and field-workers were gratified to see outbreak after outbreak contained. There were fewer surprises, hence more predictability. And as the rains came, fewer people traveled, thus slowing transmission rates.

THE BEST TIME TO WORK ON SMALLPOX IN INDIA

Even as Uttar Pradesh and Bihar were experiencing turnarounds in June, other parts of India were reporting mixed results. By May, the tally in India was four smallpox-endemic states, two troublesome states (Assam and Orissa), eight low-incidence states still bothered by importations from other areas, and sixteen states and territories that were considered smallpox free.

Madhya Pradesh looked like it might be the first of the four smallpox-endemic states to interrupt transmission. It was still reporting three to five hundred cases per month; however, the response from state health workers was good. West Bengal had seen a decrease in importations from neighboring Bihar and Bangladesh in March 1974 and a decrease in pending outbreaks from 550 in April to 450 in May. Again taking into consideration the response of state authorities, it appeared that West Bengal would be the second smallpox-endemic state to interrupt transmission.

However, potentially major problems were brewing in two of the low-incidence states. Orissa was showing a rapid increase in cases, from 53 reported in January to 565 in May. The state authorities and a superb WHO epidemiologist were able to respond appropriately, and the problem was brought under control.

Assam was a different matter. The 25 cases reported in January 1974 had not caused great alarm—after all, Bihar, by May of that year, was producing that many cases in under forty minutes. However, Assam had not received the same amount of attention as the highly endemic states; now the state was having trouble with containment, and recorded new cases increased every month thereafter, reaching a peak of 1,914 in June.

Diesh and Sharma decided they needed to visit Assam and asked me to accompany them. Americans were not allowed to travel to that area of India at that time. Nevertheless, they asked me to fly with them as far as Calcutta on the chance that we could figure out a way to get me on a flight to Guwahati, the capital of Assam. Seeing this as a potential waste of time but also assuming they had a plan, I agreed.

In fact, they had no plan at all. In Calcutta they attempted to buy a ticket to Guwahati for me. The ticket agent took one look at my passport and said that he could not sell me a ticket. Then, forty-five minutes before the flight was to leave, we experienced one of those serendipities that seemed to happen with ease around Dr. Diesh. Suddenly he spotted a minister from Assam, an old friend, and he went over to talk to him.

Diesh explained the smallpox problem, introduced me as an outside expert, and presented the dilemma of getting me to Guwahati. The minister not only trusted Dr. Diesh but also happened to be married to an American. He traveled this route often, knew the agents, and had the authority to override the usual government directives. Within minutes I had a ticket to Guwahati. I was able to attend meetings in Guwahati and Shillong, see cases of smallpox, and participate in planning the response.

From mid-1974 until the end of the year was the best time to be working on smallpox in India. Once the decline began, it was dramatic. In July, three states—Bihar, Uttar Pradesh, and West Bengal—reported 95 percent of all smallpox cases in India, with Bihar accounting for two thirds of them. But with Bihar containing over eight hundred outbreaks a week in May and June, the totals of pending outbreaks in India fell rapidly, from a peak of over eight thousand in May to fewer than six thousand in July.

Yet even as the smallpox program was finally showing obvious success, there were still attacks on the surveillance/containment strategy. Most of them involved people voicing criticism or doubt in talks or in conversations with the intent of undermining confidence, and they could be ignored. On occasion an attack was significant. In August 1974, J. B. Shrivastav, India's director-general of health services, once again lobbied the minister of health, Dr. Karan Singh, to convince him that despite the apparent success, ultimately the strategy could not work and the country was accepting great risk by discontinuing mass vaccination activities. The minister, now concerned, traveled to Bihar, still the state with by far the largest percentage of smallpox, to declare a return to mass vaccination at a press conference—this at a time when we thought we had an agreement to continue surveillance/containment and were excited about the positive results.

The minister was met at the airport in Patna by Dutta and Sharma. He told them that India did not need an "imported" strategy for smallpox, and that at the press conference he would announce that India would now return to the traditional mass vaccination campaign. Courage comes in many packages, and it was evident that day when Mahendra Dutta said if the minister wanted to do that he would have to fire Dutta first.

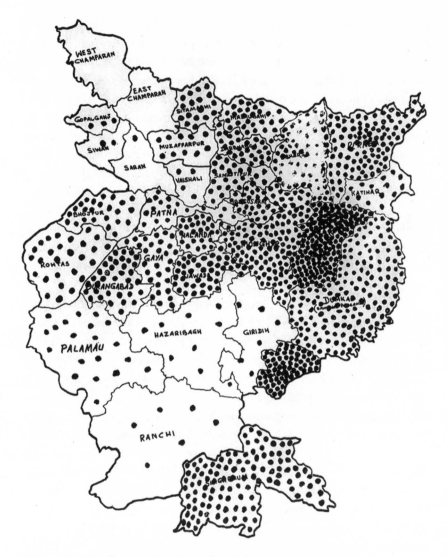

Map 3. New smallpox outbreaks in Bihar, India, 1974 and 1975 compared.
Left: New outbreaks detected in the fourth search, January 28–February 2, 1974.
Right: New outbreaks detected in the sixteenth search, January 27–February 1, 1975.

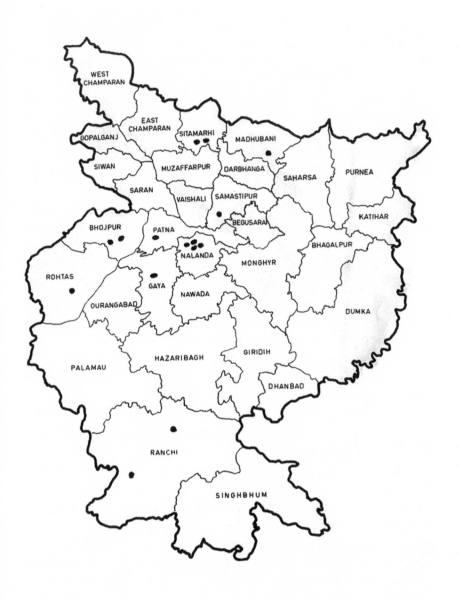

The minister responded, "Do you realize you are speaking to a minister?" Dutta replied that yes he did, but this issue was so important that he could not remain silent.[1]

The minister, surprised, listened to their account of the geographic areas that had become free of smallpox in the previous two months and the rapid progress in all districts of Bihar. To his credit, he trusted their briefing. He proceeded to the press conference, where he thanked the health workers of Bihar for the great work they were doing. He never mentioned mass vaccination. One more threat had passed.

Another followed on its heels, however. Three weeks later, Shrivastav himself, dismayed that the minister had failed to heed his warning, traveled to Bihar to make a final effort to reverse the strategy. He talked about the dangers that the backlog of children not vaccinated during the past year presented to the country. Dutta, Sharma, and Achari told him they would focus on the backlog but only after the transmission of smallpox had been broken in Bihar. (In fact, once transmission had ceased, the push for vaccinating the backlog disappeared.)

Also in August, a WHO meeting was held in New Delhi to share the smallpox eradication results from all countries in Southeast Asia. At one point, the teams from each country were invited to give their predictions for the coming months and estimate the date for the last case in their country. Speaking on behalf of the India team, I summarized India's situation, including the value of the evaluation program for predicting how fast surveillance/containment practices were improving by district. Based on the evaluation data, we were predicting that the last case of smallpox in India would be detected in May 1975. At the end of that day's meeting, workers from other countries questioned me privately. They could understand, they said, the need for optimism to keep morale high, but they were curious about my "real guess." In fact, I was completely serious about the evaluation scheme's prognostic abilities, which was now based on many months of experience. The prediction turned out to be accurate.

The work became easier as it became more predictable. With fewer surprises, the approach became one of overkill in both surveillance and containment. Nor was this the time to determine minimum inputs needed or assess maximum efficiencies across various approaches. Instead, having worked so hard to get to the current position, everyone now went overboard. Much of the work was of low efficiency. Indeed, much of it was redundant, some outright unproductive, but we were in no mood to take chances. Watch guards at each smallpox house were doubled, and searches were repeated. The vaccination circle gradually increased from the infected household itself to surrounding houses and then the entire village. Over one thousand outbreaks per month were being removed from the pending numbers for the country as a whole. The system was becoming more efficient at the same time as the size of the problem was decreasing. Madhya Pradesh, the largest state in India, had gone three weeks without a new case of smallpox. West Bengal was down to fourteen active outbreaks. Nevertheless, the high-transmission season was about to begin, and the New Delhi leadership team was especially worried about Assam, in the northeast, which had sixty-seven pending outbreaks.

By November the number of pending outbreaks in India was below one thousand. Success was becoming a tangible possibility if the disease did not get out of control during the upcoming transmission season.

Repeatedly during the campaign (and even after successfully eliminating the disease), smallpox workers received reports claiming that the disease was still present in remote populations or in groups that had been overlooked. Every such report was taken seriously and investigated, and in every instance the report was shown to be inaccurate. Often an outbreak of chicken pox or some other rash disease had been mistaken for smallpox.

Finally, the ultimate search tool was deployed. As the number of cases declined, India began to offer a reward for the reporting of previously unknown cases of smallpox. SIDA funds were used for this innovation. The reward started small, at Rs. 10 (less than US $1.50), but even that amount was large enough to cause immediate problems. When new cases were reported to health workers, the health workers wanted to claim the reward themselves. The problem was solved by providing the reward to both the person who made the report and the health worker who forwarded the report. The health worker could not claim the reward until the informant had been identified.

Initially, people tried moving smallpox patients from an outbreak area to a different village in order to collect the reward, but investigators could quickly determine that the patient was not a member of that community. No reward was paid, and people soon gave up on the idea. As the number of cases declined, the reward was increased incrementally until, at about the time of India's last cases, the reward had been increased to US$1,000.

The reward was advertised, and the general public was quick to recognize the potential bounty. Surveys were conducted to determine the percentage of people who knew about the reward and about where to report a suspected case of smallpox to collect the reward. One survey late in the campaign revealed that more people knew about the smallpox reward than knew the name of the prime minister.

OPERATION SMALLPOX ZERO

Surveillance reports for the last months of 1974 showed continuing gains. Even in Bihar, the number of new cases fell to 2,758 in October; 1,053 in November; and 527 in December. In terms of outbreaks, the year ended with only 282 pending outbreaks in all of India, and only six states reporting any smallpox cases at all. A total of twenty-four states and territories were now considered smallpox free. The investigation of outbreaks had determined that they could all be traced to human error in searches or containment. We now had an understanding of every chain of transmission in the country, and any surprises were due to the shortcomings of the workers, not a lack of understanding of the strength of the virus.

By late 1974, the smallpox program was looking so strong that it seemed very unlikely that anything could derail it. The May 1975 prediction for interruption of transmission still seemed accurate, so Paula and I began planning for our return to Atlanta in March.

A new intensification of the eradication program started in January 1975, under the code name "Operation Smallpox Zero." Six points were considered essential:

1. Every new outbreak must be visited not only by a special epidemiologist and PHC, district, and state authorities, but also by a central government or WHO officer.

2. The size of a containment team will be increased to at least twenty workers.

3. Four watch guards will be assigned to every infected house so that there will be no break in coverage.

4. House-to-house searches, in addition to the usual monthly searches, will now be undertaken in a ten-mile radius around outbreaks.

5. Laboratory specimens will be taken from one or two patients per outbreak in order to isolate the virus.

6. Cross-notification to other PHCs will occur by special messenger to avoid the delay of using the postal service.

Clearly, much of this was inefficient and made little practical sense, but like Lawrence Atutu Ochelebe, who beat the snake that entered our house in Africa to an unrecognizable pulp, we practiced overkill with smallpox, showing no mercy. The smallpox virus had met its match.

By the end of January, the number of pending outbreaks in India had declined to 198. A month later that number was 147. The week ending February 22, only 16 new outbreaks were found in the entire country, the lowest level ever recorded. The smallpox team celebrated that record, only to have it eclipsed the following week with only 3 new outbreaks found. Before going to India, I had promised Dave Sencer, in consultation with Paula, that I would be gone from the CDC for one year and would not ask for an extension. It was agonizing to see the year evaporate, but in mid-1974 Dave, knowing what the program meant to both of us, offered to extend my time. We felt bound to the original agreement, though, and so left in March, with mixed feelings. We would not have left if any doubts remained about a speedy end to smallpox in India. On the other hand, we would miss being there for the last case. In the end, we concluded there would be no program benefits to our remaining.

We left India in March, each of us knowing in our own way that we had experienced a highlight of our lives. I had been immersed in helping to solve a problem of great importance, working alongside people of

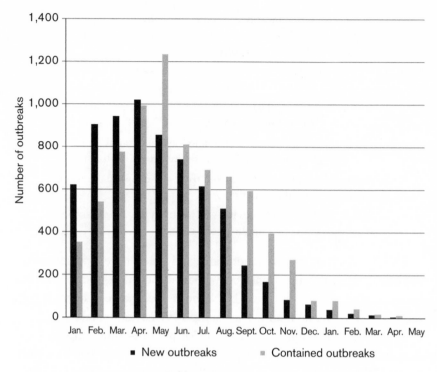

Figure 15. Total outbreaks per week in India, January 1974 to May 1975

superb abilities and motivations. The hardships were overshadowed by the blessings, and I wondered if I would ever again have the opportunity to work with people of such exceptional character.

The last case was reported in May. And on June 12, 1975, Nicole Grasset was able to send a letter to all smallpox workers in the country to say that smallpox transmission had been broken the previous month.

It seemed almost anticlimactic. A virus that for millennia had spread such despair, inspiring religious ritual and even the worship of a goddess, was suddenly gone from the country. In twenty months, the surveillance/containment approach had proved itself ideally suited for eradicating a virus that had eluded the best efforts of mass vaccination programs for 175 years. It was the right tool for the task.

THE ERADICATION OF SMALLPOX WORLDWIDE

India was one of the toughest chapters in the global fight against small-pox, but victory over smallpox in India was not the end of the story. As the last cases of smallpox were being subdued in India, Bangladesh workers were in the middle of a nightmare.

Earlier, the program in Bangladesh had been ahead of the program in India, and this information had even been used to encourage Indian workers at state meetings. In October 1974, as India still struggled with almost 1,000 outbreaks, Bangladesh had only 91 outbreaks on the books. But that month, a flood in Bangladesh, the worst in decades, decimated entire villages. People left their homes in search of food, relief, and shelter. The smallpox virus went with them, and by the end of January the outbreak count had increased from 91 to 572. This problem, already of enormous proportions, was then made worse when the government bulldozed urban slums, sending tens of thousands of refugees from urban areas to other parts of the country. The president of Bangladesh declared a national emergency.

The international community responded, not least because as more countries became free of smallpox, the importance of each infected country increased. The CDC provided thirty epidemiologists, and thirty others were sent from twenty other countries. Rewards were advertised, and a massive response to each outbreak was launched. It worked. Cases decreased through the summer. On October 16, 1975, the first vesicles of Asia's final case of smallpox began to form on a two-year-old Bangladeshi girl, Rahima Banu.

Yet globally the fight still wasn't over. As Rahima Banu was recovering, a single country, Ethiopia, remained on the smallpox list. Ethiopia had been off to a slow start. Variola minor, the strain of smallpox in Ethiopia, had a low mortality rate, and therefore smallpox was not regarded as a significant problem. Moreover, government attention had been on the political unrest that would eventually result in the overthrow of the monarchy in 1976. But now, as the last country with smallpox, Ethiopia could no longer ignore the problem. WHO helped arrange for supplies, helicopters, and several dozen foreign advisors. By early

1976, after a herculean effort, the country had become free of smallpox except for an area in the Blue Nile Gorge and in the desert of the south. By August, Ethiopia had eliminated the last cases.

It seemed to be time for the world to celebrate. But Murphy's Law (anything that can go wrong will go wrong) operates no less frequently in public health programs than elsewhere. At the last moment the tenacity of this virus, combined with the movement of people, again intervened. Drought in the south forced some Ethiopians to seek refuge in Somalia. In September 1976, smallpox cases were reported in Mogadishu, Somalia's capital. Six months later, outbreaks were occurring around the country. National and international resources descended on the problem areas. Two dozen WHO epidemiologists and thousands of Somalian health workers carried out the now-familiar surveillance/containment procedures under what some consider the most difficult conditions of a hard decade. Again the strategy worked.

In early October 1977, a couple with two small children, both with smallpox, approached the hospital in Merka, Somalia. They asked Ali Maow Maalin, an employee, for directions to the infectious disease ward. A considerate person, he took them to the ward rather than directing them. Although he had been vaccinated, it was evidently not an effective take. Two weeks later, on October 26, 1977, he developed the last smallpox rash that Africa would ever see. He recovered without transmitting the virus. The global chain of smallpox transmission was finally broken. Smallpox had been eliminated from the world because of a plan. It did not happen by accident.

There was yet a final irony. After ten months of worldwide freedom from smallpox, the country that had provided the vaccine to the world had two final cases. Both were due to a virus that escaped from a laboratory—demonstrating again the challenge of containing this tenacious virus. On August 11, 1978, a woman in Birmingham, England, developed the first symptoms of smallpox and died a month later. Her mother developed symptoms on September 2, 1978, but recovered.[2]

In medicine, the medical practitioner is obliged to apply the best knowledge of the times to each patient. In public health, the obligation is to apply the best knowledge to the entire human community. The purpose of public health is to promote social justice. By 1978, public health achieved its first complete success in social justice, applying the knowledge required for smallpox control to eliminate a disease for current humanity and for all future generations. Humanity will continue to hold its collective breath, hoping for the wisdom that prevents the virus from ever being released again—intentionally or unintentionally.

Conclusion

The smallpox program justified its own existence by the results it produced: lives set free, misery prevented, and resources made available for other activities. The program also offers lessons that are applicable to similar public health projects.[1]

Smallpox eradication did not happen by accident. Stephen Hawking, in his book *A Brief History of Time,* says the history of science is the gradual realization that things do not happen in an arbitrary fashion. This is a cause-and-effect world, and smallpox disappeared because of a plan, conceived and implemented on purpose, by people. Humanity does not have to live in a world of plagues, disastrous governments, conflict, and uncontrolled health risks. The coordinated action of a group of dedicated people can plan for and bring about a better future. The fact of smallpox eradication remains a constant reminder that we should settle for nothing less.

Seek the truth. The purpose of surveillance systems is to discover the truth. Once the truth was known concerning where the smallpox virus was at a given point in time, it was possible to eliminate it. The strategy of mass vaccination is founded on the assumption that it is not possible to know where a virus is. Therefore one must assume that it could be anyplace, and the appropriate response is to protect everyone to achieve herd immunity. That logic works with most infectious diseases, but not with smallpox.

Every earlier review of the smallpox problem in India recommended high vaccination coverage of every segment of the population. Experts from India, from WHO, and from the CDC all concluded that since 80 percent coverage was not being achieved, the goal needed to be increased to 100 percent. That makes no sense. If you can't reach 80 percent, you certainly can't reach 100 percent. The herd immunity concept was promoted yet remained unexamined.

Knowledge is power, and even a little knowledge of the truth goes a long way. Even less-than-perfect surveillance in the early months of the new strategy, October to December 1973, followed by poor containment efforts, was still relatively effective in reducing virus transmission. Once surveillance and containment reached near perfection in May 1974, the result was a rapid decline from extremely high levels of smallpox to zero smallpox in twelve months. This is a feat unprecedented in public health history.

However, the truth that we came to know about smallpox is not necessarily the truth about other diseases. What is true is that each particular disease and its context must to studied in order to understand its vulnerabilities. Mass vaccination continues to be an important strategy for most vaccine-preventable diseases.

Spend the time and attention needed to systematically improve the tools as well as the techniques to deliver them. WHO developed a better vaccine and adopted a superior vaccination technique, the bifurcated needle, both of which were essential to success. The program was also constantly refining the techniques used to efficiently track the virus and to encircle the virus with people immune to smallpox.

Coalitions are powerful. Successful coalitions share certain characteristics, the first being a clear vision of the last mile of the journey, which in this case was the total absence of smallpox cases and smallpox transmission. Yet the secret to the eradication of smallpox in India was that the members of the coalition team suppressed their individual egos for the sake of achieving a common goal. Moreover, the boundaries between the Central Government, the states, the districts, WHO, NGOs, public institutions, and private industry were obscured as the team formed with an unwavering focus on the desired outcome. This was clear to participants, yet has been missed by some recent historians.

Trust holds teams together. It was trust that allowed for transparent discussion and productive arguments about tactics. It was trust in Drs. Mahendra Dutta and M. I. D. Sharma that allowed Dr. Karan Singh, India's minister of health, to support surveillance/containment when others were advising him to return to mass vaccination.

Social will is crucial. Individual will leads people to seek the protection of vaccines, but it is the collective will that drives individuals to provide resources and opportunities for others to be protected. Government support for programs depends on the agreement of the governed. In theory, eradicating smallpox was possible from the time vaccine became available. It became easier as science and technology improved the tools and delivery techniques. But that was not enough. The 1970s became the last decade for smallpox because of social will—a collective agreement to remove the scourge from society.

Social will must be transformed into political will. Every public health decision ultimately requires a political decision for implementation. Therefore, public health practitioners must provide politicians with the information needed for good public policy decisions.

Public health solutions rest on good science, but the implementation of those practices depends on good management. Smallpox posed some intriguing scientific problems, but eradication depended on the managers. Countries often insisted that the consultants had to be physicians even if they were less effective in running field programs.[2] In both Africa and India, people trained in program management were extremely valuable.

Tactical flexibility is crucial. Workers were encouraged to experiment with tactical approaches, which if effective could readily be replicated by other workers. Monthly meetings in every endemic state allowed for rapid transfer of information. We didn't wait for annual reviews. Monthly meetings allowed us to refine tools and techniques as quickly as we could get information from surveillance and evaluations.

Allocate resources where they are needed. It is crucial to have the ability to concentrate all available skills and resources on the point of need. In the words of a young Indian physician, "Put water on the house that is burning rather than on the other houses."

Effective leadership is crucial. The smallpox eradication program benefited immensely from effective leadership. Key in this area were unflagging dedication to the program's objectives, an ongoing willingness to use new information to improve the strategy, and the capacity to build coalitions.

Never give up. Tenacity won't always bring success, but without it, success is impossible.

The measure of civilization is how people treat each other. How people treat each other is the metric for a civilized nation, political party, society, university, or program. How we treat each other is also the measure of us as individuals. The smallpox eradication program was a civilized program in that it transformed potential smallpox patients into immune persons and protected unseen people in the generations to come.

Be optimistic. The trouble with being an optimist, of course, is that people think you don't know what's going on. But it is the way to live. We were an optimistic group. I tell students there is a place for pessimism, and whenever they need it, they should contract for it—but don't put those people on their payroll. They will ruin your day.

Global efforts are possible. The smallpox eradication effort proved that it is possible to choose a global objective and bring global resources to bear on it. Philosopher Will Durant once observed that the world was unlikely to join forces unless it feared an alien invasion. Smallpox demonstrated that problems short of an alien invasion can mobilize the world. Smallpox was a shared risk, and its removal required a shared effort. In the years since then, other problems—nuclear arms, polio, SARS, HIV, H1N1 flu (surrogates for an alien invasion)—have confirmed the power of understanding shared risks. Pursuing such problems is worth the effort both because of the inherent good in solving them and because they provide practice in working together and breaking down unnecessary and unproductive social barriers.

The objective may be global, but implementation is always local. The strategy for smallpox eradication did not change from country to country, but the local culture determined which tactics were most useful. Only the specific locality can provide information on who is sick, who is hiding from the vaccinators, when people are available for vaccination, how to hire watch guards, or how to secure the cooperation of the community. In all cultures, an approach of respect for local customs is needed.

Communications functions as the nervous system of successful coalitions. Efforts to report from the search and containment workers to the PHC, then to the district, the state, and finally the central level improved continuously. The surveillance reports were collated and analyzed, and the results were shared widely through the systemic feedback, all the way back to the PHC staff doing the work. Local workers knew their position in the global effort. "We are all in this together" was a palpable feeling. This in turn engendered a pride in the work being done. Trust, effectiveness, and knowing the truth all depended on good communication systems.

Effective evaluation methods are key to success. Evaluation was the key to identifying and remediating deficiencies in the strategy. Evaluation was also crucial to knowing when each district and state would reach the tipping point of controlling smallpox faster than it was spreading. Evaluation made it possible to predict where resources were needed in advance rather than simply reacting to the information of the day. It was not an add-on; evaluation was a priority management tool that helped make effective use of scarce resources. The mantra from the American Management Association was repeated hundreds of times: "You get what you inspect, not what you expect."

Humility does not mean fatalism. In retrospect, achieving the eradication of smallpox might look inevitable. In fact, though, the chain of events included so many opportunities for failure that success was not a given— and we knew it. We had no guarantee of success and were humbled so often that humility became a daily emotion. *We didn't let that stop us.*

Postscript

Over the years, on every return to India, I have
searched the faces of people on the street, looking
for pockmarks. Soon I could find no pockmarked
face under the age of ten, then twenty, and now,
no pockmarks are to be found on people under
the age of thirty-five.

A Plan in the Event of
Smallpox Bioterrorism

In 2002, the United States was concerned that Iraq might have weaponized the smallpox virus, and the U.S. government quickly moved to set up a prevention program. Crucial lessons from the global smallpox program seemed to be totally forgotten or ignored. The rather anemic response was a plan to vaccinate first responders, then medical personnel, and finally, in the event of smallpox, to vaccinate 10 million people in ten days.

Moreover, the public health leadership seemed to be oblivious to the potential for a complete breakdown of the social order. Even a single case of smallpox in the United States would have resulted in panic, with 300 million people demanding vaccination immediately, fighting to be part of the initial vaccination cohort.

Lessons learned from the global smallpox eradication effort could be used to formulate a technically sound plan that would ensure the quick containment of dozens, even hundreds, of simultaneous outbreaks in the United States, and to communicate that plan to the public:

1. Emphasize to the public that anyone vaccinated on the day of exposure or even within three days after exposure will be protected from the disease. Describe how a dozen or even a hundred outbreaks could be contained with relative ease. (The problems would come if many hundreds of outbreaks became apparent at one time. That would require the capacity for mass vaccination.)

2. Present the details of how everyone in this country could be vaccinated within three days, even in a worst-case scenario with thousands of cases discovered simultaneously throughout the country.

3. Decentralize the vaccination program to each of the three thousand counties in the country.

4. Designate every high school as a vaccination site, since people usually know the high school district they live in.

5. Calculate the number of people living in the catchment area of each high school to determine the number of vaccinations and therefore the number of vaccinators required to vaccinate everyone in three days.

6. Recruit in advance medical personnel, teachers, government workers, and volunteers to perform the vaccinations. The technique can be taught in fifteen minutes. A practice session in advance and a refresher session on the first day of vaccinations would be sufficient.

7. Plan to run the vaccination clinics twenty-four hours a day until everyone has been vaccinated. The procedure is so easy that the number of vaccinators could even be doubled so complete vaccination could be accomplished in two days, if needed.

8. Keep the vaccine in a central location, if there is concern about storage conditions, with advance plans to ship the vaccine overnight to each of the three thousand counties. Containers for shipping could be available; address labels could be affixed in advance.

This plan, using the lessons learned during the global program, would quickly contain dozens, even hundreds, of simultaneous outbreaks in the United States. Informing the public of the plan would prevent uncontrollable panic.

INSTRUCTIONS FOR SMALLPOX VACCINATION WITH BIFURCATED NEEDLE

1. Method for vaccination with the bifurcated needle – MULTIPUNCTURE technique.
2. Site of vaccination – outer aspect of upper arm over the insertion of deltoid muscle.
3. Preparation of skin – none.   If site is obviously dirty, a cloth moistened with water may be used to wipe the site.
4. Withdrawal of vaccine from ampoule.   A sterile bifurcated needle (which must be cool if flamed or completely dry if boiled) is inserted into the ampoule of reconstituted vaccine. On withdrawal, a droplet of vaccine, sufficient for vaccination is contained within the fork of the needle.
5. Application of vaccine to the skin.   The needle is held at a 90° angle (perpendicular) to the skin.   (See figure.)   The wrist of the vaccinator rests against the arm.   The points are touched lightly to the skin surface permitting the droplet of vaccine to be deposited on the skin.   For both primovaccination and revaccination, 15 up and down (perpendicular) strokes of the needle are rapidly made in the area of about 5 mm in diameter (through the drop of vaccine deposited on the skin).   The strokes should be sufficiently vigorous so that a trace of blood appears at the vaccination site.   If a trace of blood does not appear, the strokes have not been sufficiently vigorous and the procedure should be repeated.   Although it is desirable not to induce frank bleeding, the proportion of successful takes is not reduced if bleeding does occur.
6. No dressing should be used after vaccination.
7. Sterilization of needle may be done by flaming or boiling.
   (a) Flaming – the needle is passed through the flame of a spirit lamp.   It should not remain in the flame for more than 3 seconds.   The needle must be allowed to cool completely before inserting into vaccine ampoule.
   (b) Boiling – the needle is sterilized by boiling for 20 minutes.   Subsequently, the needle must be dried thoroughly to ensure that the fork of the needle does not contain a drop of water when inserted into the vaccine ampoule.
8. Unused, reconstituted freeze-dried vaccine should be discarded at the end of each working day.

MULTIPUNCTURE VACCINATION BY BIFURCATED NEEDLE

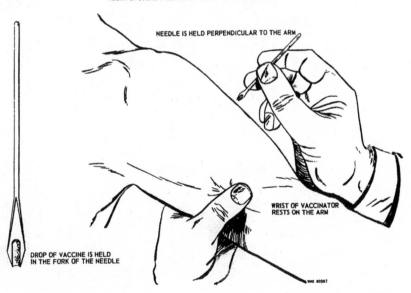

NEEDLE IS HELD PERPENDICULAR TO THE ARM

WRIST OF VACCINATOR
RESTS ON THE ARM

DROP OF VACCINE IS HELD
IN THE FORK OF THE NEEDLE

WHO 80567

Figure 16. Instructions given to field-workers for vaccinating with the bifurcated needle

Notes

ONE. A LOATHSOME DISEASE

1. Donald R. Hopkins, *Princes and Peasants: Smallpox in History* (Chicago: University of Chicago Press, 1983).

2. Donald R. Hopkins, personal communication, December 1979.

3. G. Catlin, *O-Kee-Pa, a Religious Ceremony, and Other Customs of the Mandans* (1867. Centennial edition, edited by J.C. Ewers, New Haven, CT: Yale University Press, 1967).

4. Elizabeth A. Fenn, *Pox Americana: The Great Smallpox Epidemic of 1775–82* (New York: Hill and Wang, 2001).

5. Garry Wills, *Lincoln at Gettysburg: The Words That Remade America* (New York: Simon and Schuster, 1992).

6. Hopkins, *Princes and Peasants*.

7. Edward Jenner, *An Inquiry into the Causes and Effects of the Variolae Vaccinae, a Disease Discovered in Some of the Western Counties of England, Particularly Gloucestershire, and Known by the Name of the Cowpox* (1798. Reprint, Denver, CO: Nolie Mumey, 1940).

8. Jefferson quoted in Hopkins, *Princes and Peasants*, 310.

TWO. A SUCCESSION OF MENTORS

1. Some years later, Ravenholt's interest in global fertility control led him to head up the population program at the U.S. Agency for International Development (USAID). For a compilation of Ravenholt's contributions, see "Adventures in Epidemiology," January 15, 2009, at www.ravenholt.com.

2. Through the years, the name changed first to Center for Disease Control, then to Centers for Disease Control, and finally to Centers for Disease Control and Prevention. The acronym (CDC) remains unchanged.

3. For more information, see "Epidemic Intelligence Service," www.cdc.gov/eis/, accessed December 14, 2008.

4. C. W. Dixon, *Smallpox* (London: J. and A. Churchill Ltd., 1962).

5. W. H. Foege, "Investigation of Suspected Smallpox—New Mexico," Report to J. D. Millar, March 1963. Archives housed in the Epidemic Intelligence Service, Centers for Disease Control and Prevention, Atlanta, Georgia (hereafter cited as CDC Files).

6. Jim Curran, *K2: The Story of the Savage Mountain* (Seattle: The Mountaineers, 1995); Robert H. Bates and Charles S. Houston, *Five Miles High: The Story of an Attack on the Second Highest Mountain in the World by the Members of the First American Karakoram Expedition*, 2nd ed. (New York: Lyons Press, 2000).

7. T. H. Weller, "Questions of Priority," *New England Journal of Medicine* 269 (1963): 673-78.

8. Tom Weller, John Enders, and Fred Robbins had won a Nobel Prize in 1954 for demonstrating that it is possible to grow poliovirus under laboratory conditions, thereby setting the stage for the development of polio vaccine, which was licensed in 1955. Weller remained active and interested in global health for the rest of his life. He died in 2008 at the age of ninety-four.

9. F. Fenner, D. A. Henderson, I. Arita, and Z. Jezek, *Smallpox and Its Eradication* (Geneva: World Health Organization, 1988), 409.

10. Rei Ravenholt to Sargent Shriver, June 24, 1961. Author's personal files.

THREE. PRACTICING PUBLIC HEALTH IN NIGERIA

1. Personal communication, June 1965.

2. See, for instance, S. Bhattacharya, M. Harrison, and M. Worboys, *Fractured States: Smallpox, Public Health, and Vaccination Policy in British India 1800–1947* (New Delhi: Orient Longman, 2005).

3. Elenore Smith Bowen [Laura Bohannan], *Return to Laughter: An Anthropological Novel* (Garden City, NY: Doubleday, 1964), 230.

4. Ibid., 231–44.

5. William Schneider, "Smallpox in Africa during Colonial Rule," *Medical History* 53 (2009).

6. Ibid.

7. Donald R. Hopkins, *Princes and Peasants: Smallpox in History* (Chicago: University of Chicago Press, 1983).

8. Hausa woman quoted in Schneider, "Smallpox in Africa during Colonial Rule," 198.

FOUR. FIRE LINE AROUND A VIRUS

1. The program was staffed by over three dozen unique workers. One example is Dr. George Lythcott, a pediatrician who headed up the regional office established by CDC in Lagos, Nigeria. He displayed exceptional interpersonal skills that often made the difference in getting African authorities to agree to the program and to any needed changes. Stories abounded of his fast and intuitive responses, and as an African American he seemed to get an immediate and positive response from Africans at all levels. In one country, when he was unable to see the head of state to get an agreement signed, he reportedly contacted the man's mistress, who arranged for a meeting and a signature. In West Africa, while he was escorting the surgeon general in a celebration of the 25 millionth smallpox vaccination, a sudden change of plans required an unexpected stop in Togo. George's visa had expired, but he was not about to be left behind. He had no idea how he was going to get admitted to the country. With the help of one of the French-speaking CDC people, he practiced some phrases to use on the immigration officer, who surely would understand his predicament. At the immigration counter, he was totally surprised to be greeted by a young Togolese woman. Forgetting the French phrases, he adopted a different persona, greeting her with, "Hi, Baby!" He then asked if he could "borrow her Bic," and in front of her, with her pen, he changed the date on his expired visa. She was suitably charmed, stamped his visa, and once again George successfully made up the rules on the fly.

George would immediately get to know the people in an office, at the airport, or in the field. One time in the departure area at the Lagos airport, having made his usual rounds, he came back to me saying, "They have overbooked by three people. If they call your name for a phone call do not go to the other room." Minutes later, three names were announced; they had phone calls. Would they please go to the next room and identify themselves? Three people left the room, the door closed, and the airline immediately boarded the rest of us. On another flight, George learned that some first-class seats would be empty. He offered to show me how to travel first class on the condition that I kept my mouth shut and let him do all of the negotiating. We walked to the first-class section and sat down. George made it a point to go to the cockpit just to say to the pilot, "It is good to see you again." The flight attendant now thought they were friends. Later, she looked at his ticket and said, "I am sorry, this is a coach ticket." George looked surprised and said, "Certainly you won't discriminate against me because I don't have enough money for a first-class ticket." Thinking he was the pilot's friend, she let him stay. Looking at my ticket, she started to tell me I couldn't stay in first class, but George just brushed it off, saying, "He's with me."

A few years later, George and I were sent to Calabar after it was captured by the federal troops during the Nigerian Civil War. The embassy had asked us to do a survey of the condition of children in the area. As we were leaving Lagos in a Nigerian military aircraft loaded with fifty-five gallon drums of jet fuel and oxygen tanks, in a lightning storm, George said, "Do you realize traveling on a military plane to a war area means our life insurance is no good?" He continued, "I can't take this. I'm going to sleep." Which he did. On arrival in Calabar, a military jeep took us to the commanding officer, who told us where we would sleep and eat, and how we would use a military jeep to do our survey. As we were leaving he asked, "Do you want women for the night?" George, never lost for words, said, "Thanks anyway, but my friend here is a preacher."

2. F. Fenner, D. A Henderson, I. Arita, and Z. Jezek, *Smallpox and Its Eradication* (Geneva: World Health Organization, 1988), 903.

3. Ibid.

FIVE. EXTINGUISHING SMALLPOX IN A TIME OF WAR

1. Peter Enahoro, *How to Be a Nigerian* (Santa Rosa, CA: Spectrum Books Ltd., 1998), 21.

2. World Health Organization, *Smallpox Eradication—Report of a WHO Scientific Group*, Technical Report Series no. 383 (Geneva: WHO, 1968).

3. W. H. Foege, "Epidemiology of Smallpox in West and Central Africa," Seminar on Smallpox Eradication and Measles Control in Western and Central Africa (Lagos, Nigeria, May 13–20, 1969).

4. Henry M. Gelfand and D. A. Henderson, "A Program for Smallpox Eradication and Measles Control throughout West Africa," *Journal of International Health* 2, no. 1 (Fall 1966).

5. CDC, *West and Central African Smallpox Eradication/Measles Control Program—Manual of Operations*, issued October 1, 1966. The author of the manual is not identified in the manual itself. However, in an interview published as "Smallpox: Dispelling the Myths" (*Bulletin of the World Health Organization* 86, no. 12, December 2008), D. A. Henderson states that he and others prepared the

manual for West and Central Africa; Henderson then modified it for other parts of the world.

6. CDC, *West and Central African Smallpox Eradication.*

SIX. UNDER THE RULE OF VARIOLA

1. Letter from H. Gelfand to J. D. Millar, May 2, 1969. Author's personal files.

2. F. Fenner, D. A. Henderson, I. Arita, and Z. Jezek, *Smallpox and Its Eradication* (Geneva: World Health Organization, 1988).

3. J. Z. Holwell, "An Account of the Manner of Inoculating for Smallpox in the East Indies (AD 1767)," in *Indian Science and Technology in the Eighteenth Century: Some Contemporary European Accounts,* vol. 1 of *Collected Writings of Dharampal* (Delhi: Impex, 1971), 143–63.

4. My thanks to Dr. M. I. D. Sharma for his help in assembling the following material on smallpox in India.

5. G. Mukhopadhya, *History of Indian Medicine,* 2nd ed. (New Delhi: Oriental Books Reprint Corporation, 1974).

6. O. P. Jaggi, *Folk Medicine* (Delhi: Atma Ram and Sons, 1973).

7. S. Bhattacharya, M. Harrison, and M. Worboys, *Fractured States: Smallpox, Public Health and Vaccination Policy in British India 1800–1947* (New Delhi: Orient Longman, 2005), 64.

8. Holwell, "Account of the Manner of Inoculating for Smallpox."

9. C. W. Dixon, *Smallpox* (London: J. and A. Churchill Ltd., 1962); K. M. Lal, D. Chand, and G. S. Murty, "Smallpox in Uttar Pradesh (1877–1954)," *Journal of the Indian Medical Association* 30, no. 4 (1958): 120–26.

10. M. I. D. Sharma, *The History of Smallpox in India,* unpublished paper, 1980. Author's personal files.

11. *British Medical Journal,* Jenner Centenary Number, May 23, 1896.

12. Donald R. Hopkins, *Princes and Peasants: Smallpox in History* (Chicago: University of Chicago Press, 1983), 74.

13. S. P. James, *Smallpox and Vaccination in British India* (Calcutta: Thacker, Spink and Co., 1909).

14. Sharma, *History of Smallpox in India.*

15. R. W. Hunter, *A Statistical Account of Bengal* (London: Trubner and Co., 1876).

16. S. J. Thompson, *The Silent India* (Edinburgh: Williams, Blackwood and Sons, 1913).

17. Bhattacharya, Harrison, and Worboys, *Fractured States,* 35.

18. Ibid., 54.

19. Hopkins, *Princes and Peasants,* 147–48. S. J. Thompson reports that simi-

lar rumors were repeated in Burma as part of an antivaccination campaign. See Thompson, *Silent India*.

20. Bhattacharya, Harrison, and Worboys, *Fractured States*.

21. James, *Smallpox and Vaccination in British India*.

22. Bhattacharya, Harrison, and Worboys, *Fractured States*, 64.

23. Health Survey and Development Committee, Report (Delhi: Manager of Publications, 1946).

24. R. N. Basu, Z. Jezek, and N. A. Ward, *The Eradication of Smallpox from India* (Geneva: World Health Organization, 1979).

25. *Control of Smallpox and Cholera in India. Report on the Deliberations of the Central Expert Committee of Indian Council of Medical Research on Smallpox and Cholera* (New Delhi: Ministry of Health, Government of India, 1959).

26. *National Smallpox Eradication Programme in India* (New Delhi: Ministry of Health and Family Planning, Government of India, 1966).

27. India's National Institute of Communicable Diseases is equivalent to the Centers for Disease Control and Prevention in the United States; indeed it was renamed the National Centre for Disease Control at its centennial celebration in July 2009. See K. C. Patnaik and P. N. Kapoor, *Statistical Review of Smallpox Problem in India* (New Delhi: Central Bureau of Health Intelligence, 1965); H. M. Gelfand, "A Critical Examination of the Indian Smallpox Eradication Program," *American Journal of Public Health and the Nation's Health* 56, no. 10 (1966): 1634–51; S. P. Ramakrishnan and H. M Gelfand, *A Guide for the Evaluation of the National Smallpox Eradication Programme at the District Level* (New Delhi: Government of India, Ministry of Health, 1964).

28. World Health Organization, "An Assessment of the National Smallpox Eradication Programme," restricted report (Geneva: WHO, 1968).

29. The jet injector was awkward to transport, required setting up and taking down at each stop, and was expensive to purchase and maintain. In May 1967, a team headed by Dr. Ralph (Rafe) Henderson tried unsuccessfully to introduce jet injectors into India. Rafe Henderson was working in the smallpox regional office in Lagos, Nigeria, and his team included Drs. Lyle Conrad and Gordon Reid from the CDC. As the team set up to demonstrate the usefulness of the jet injector by using it on Indian health officials, they discovered they had no saline diluent with them. They substituted sterile water, which can be used as a diluent with no reduction in vaccination take rates. Unlike the diluent, however, sterile water causes significant stinging at the injection site. The CDC team successfully demonstrated how easy it was to use the jet injector, but the painful stinging left the health officials unconvinced. The team worked in both urban and rural areas to combat smallpox outbreaks, but left India frustrated because the jet injector was not widely accepted. Years afterward, Henderson learned

that initially there were high expectations that the introduction of jet injectors in India might lead to smallpox eradication in a period of weeks (Ralph Henderson, personal communication, March 2010). In West Africa years later, smallpox workers would always ship vaccine and diluent together, even if sending diluent by air was costly, in order to avoid the pain caused by using sterile water to dilute the vaccine.

30. Shortly after obtaining the patent, Wyeth waived royalties on any bifurcated needles produced under WHO auspices. This act of corporate philanthropy in global health (later known as pharmacophilanthropy) was a defining moment for the smallpox eradication effort. Pharmaceutical companies would later increase their contributions to global health dramatically. Merck, for example, provided hundreds of millions of treatments of Mectizan to prevent river blindness, and GlaxoSmithKline provided Albendazole for the global lymphatic filiarises program. Merck teamed up with the Gates Foundation to bring twenty-first-century science to Botswana, demonstrating the ability to rapidly treat HIV infections and to reduce HIV positivity in newborns by over 90 percent. Unfortunately, the public has been inadequately versed about pharmaceutical companies' recent attempts to assist in the improvement of global health. Wyeth provided early leadership.

31. S. Bhattacharya, *Expunging Variola — The Control and Eradication of Smallpox in India, 1947–1977* (New Delhi: Orient Longman, 2006), 147.

32. Ibid.

SEVEN. UNWARRANTED OPTIMISM

1. This fact was poorly understood in the debates surrounding the attempt to vaccinate U.S. citizens in 2002. Public health officials and others who had not participated in the smallpox eradication program insisted that surveillance and containment procedures could not work in the United States. Immunity levels, they argued, were extremely low on account of the cessation of routine smallpox vaccinations in the early 1970s. Given the realities of population density, however, surveillance and containment would have been less difficult in the United States than in most of the situations encountered in Bihar in 1974 because of fewer susceptible people per square mile.

2. Henry Gelfand once theorized that the sex trade probably created the ultimate transmission problem with smallpox, since prostitutes could still work early in their illness, before they realized they were sick. Indeed, some outbreak investigations supported his theory.

3. Minister of health's speech from author's personal files.

EIGHT. A GORGEOUS COALITION

1. Larry Brilliant and his wife, Girija, went on to have stellar careers in public health and the business world. They were key to developing the Seva Foundation, which focused on remediating blindness in the subcontinent. Larry later wrote a book, *The Management of Smallpox Eradication in India* (Ann Arbor: University of Michigan Press, 1985). His work culminated in his leadership of the Google philanthropy effort.

2. A. R. Rao, *Smallpox* (Bombay: Kothari Book Depot, 1972).

3. Personal communication, Don Francis, January 16, 2009.

4. S. Bhattacharya, *Expunging Variola: The Control and Eradication of Smallpox in India, 1947–1977* (New Delhi: Orient Longman, 2006).

5. The CDC West and Central Africa program attempted to augment the archives by securing oral histories from the participants who returned for the forty-year reunion of smallpox warriors in 2006, held in Atlanta. This effort was so productive that oral histories were also obtained from people working in Asia who met in Atlanta in 2008, and an archive has been established at Emory University. For more details, see http://globalhealthchronicles.org/smallpox.

NINE. RISING NUMBERS, REFINING STRATEGY

1. Coercion was never program policy. A 1995 article by Paul Greenough gives the erroneous impression that coercion was required for containment to work in the final elimination of smallpox. He recounts four instances in which two American epidemiologists used coercion plus a fifth instance in which an Indian government vaccinator used force to hold and vaccinate people. Greenough also quotes from the journal of an American smallpox worker who attempted unsuccessfully to persuade a woman to be vaccinated. The worker was ejected from the home by the woman's husband. The cases cited are no doubt true, but they would have been aberrations, perhaps the result of the kind of frustration that anyone who has worked in the field can understand. Cultural sensitivity was emphasized in the training of smallpox workers in India and in the field was the norm rather than the exception. Certainly force was not needed for eradication. Greenough interpreted this aberration to be the norm. See P. Greenough, "Intimidation, Coercion and Resistance in the Final Stages of the South Asian Smallpox Eradication Campaign, 1973–75," *Social Science and Medicine* 41, no. 5 (1995): 633–45.

2. R. N. Basu, Z. Jezek, and N. A. Ward, *The Eradication of Smallpox from India* (Geneva: World Health Organization, 1979).

TEN. WATER ON A BURNING HOUSE

1. Myron L. Belkind, *Smallpox* (New Delhi: Associated Press, 1974).
2. Letter from H. Gelfand to J. D. Millar, dated May 2, 1969. Author's personal files.
3. Report in author's personal files.

ELEVEN. SMALLPOX ZERO

1. Mahendra Dutta, personal communication, August 2, 2009.
2. F. Fenner, D. A Henderson, I. Arita, and Z. Jezek, *Smallpox and Its Eradication* (Geneva: World Health Organization, 1988), 1097.

CONCLUSION

1. This conclusion is based on a talk I gave in 2009 at the commemoration of thirty years of global freedom from smallpox held at the WHO regional headquarters in New Delhi.
2. From one standpoint, physicians are actually managers, taught to analyze a health problem in an individual, determine the objective for that person, plan a strategy to achieve the objective, monitor indicators to evaluate whether the management strategy is working, and make midcourse corrections to modify the strategy. However, physicians often miss this point and fail to apply their managerial skills beyond clinical medicine.

Glossary

CDC   Centers for Disease Control and Prevention in Atlanta, Georgia. Known in earlier years as the Communicable Disease Center, the Center for Disease Control, and the Centers for Disease Control.

containment   The response to finding a smallpox case or outbreak. The term initially referred to containing the smallpox virus so that it could not spread to others, but its meaning evolved to include a wide range of activities involving a local census, vaccination of potential contacts, watch guards at the houses of smallpox cases, etc.

EIS   Epidemic Intelligence Service, a program at CDC that recruits people for two-year terms to study and respond to disease threats of all kinds. EIS officers figured heavily in smallpox eradication.

epidemiology   The study of patterns of health, illness, and associated factors in the population as a whole.

fetisheurs   Local medicine men in West Africa who treated individuals with smallpox. They represented a mixture of medical and religious beliefs and had learned how to propagate smallpox by collecting scabs from smallpox patients and inducing new outbreaks when they desired new patients.

herd immunity   High immunity levels to a disease in a population, making it difficult or impossible for the disease agent to spread.

Indian government   The responsibility for smallpox eradication involved the Central Ministry of Health in Delhi, state governments, districts (subdivisions of states), and blocks (subdivisions of districts). Blocks were inhabited by approximately one hundred thousand people. In general, Primary Health Centers coincided with blocks, and so provided health services for one hundred thousand people.

mass vaccination   The systematic vaccination of all segments of the population in an attempt to develop herd immunity.

Nigerian government   In 1966 the responsibility for smallpox eradication involved the National Ministry of Health in Lagos and four regions: the Northern Region, the Western Region, the Midwest Region, and the Eastern Region. The regions were subdivided into provinces. Later, Nigeria was subdivided into states.

searches   The activities involved in finding cases of smallpox. Primary searches involved going through villages and urban areas looking for cases. Secondary searches were conducted at markets or festivals in an effort to obtain information on smallpox in the areas from which people had come. Tertiary searches focused on areas or populations deemed to have a high risk for smallpox cases, such as beggar communities, kiln worker communities, mobile roadway workers, etc.

SEARO   Southeast Asia Regional Office, a WHO regional office responsible for India, Bangladesh, and other countries.

smallpox outbreaks   From one to hundreds of cases in a geographic area, such as a village or a neighborhood in an urban area. *New outbreak* means an outbreak newly detected by searches or through the passive surveillance system, which would then be targeted for containment activities. *Deleted outbreak* refers to an outbreak that had now gone the requisite time without a new case of smallpox, usually four to six weeks. *Pending outbreaks* refers to all outbreaks still receiving containment attention. This category included new and active outbreaks; these remained pending until a period of no new cases had passed.

special epidemiologists   Workers from elsewhere in India or other countries who focused on problem districts to provide supervision for search and containment activities.

surveillance   The systematic monitoring of all information related to a disease, in this case smallpox. This term was often used in the restricted sense of attempting to find all cases of smallpox.

take   A successful vaccination as evidenced by the appearance of a sore, crater, or blister at the site of a vaccination several days after the vaccination.

vaccination   The act of transferring cowpox or vaccinia virus in order to induce immunity to smallpox. (Louis Pasteur later suggested that in order to honor Edward Jenner, all immunizations could be called "vaccinations" and all immunizing agents could be called "vaccines.")

vaccine   A preparation that improves immunity to a particular disease. The term *vaccine* comes from the term for cowpox (*vaccinae*). When cowpox was administered to humans, it provided protection from smallpox.

vaccinology   The field of study dealing with vaccines.

variolation   Also called *inoculation, variolation* refers to transferring smallpox virus itself from a patient with smallpox to a scratch or abrasion on a healthy person to induce immunity to smallpox. This would actually give the recipient a case of smallpox that was usually milder than if the virus had been acquired through the usual respiratory route. This practice predates vaccination by hundreds if not thousands of years. The danger was that the virus could then spread to others, causing outbreaks of smallpox.

virus   A small infectious agent unable to replicate unless it is inside the living cells of another organism. (Smallpox is spread by a virus.)

watch guards   Workers hired to stay at the homes of smallpox patients to vaccinate every person who came to visit.

WHO   World Health Organization in Geneva, Switzerland. Policy is developed through annual World Health Assembly (WHA) meetings, attended by the ministers of health of all member countries.

Index

Abakaliki, Nigeria, 58–59
Accra, Ghana, 69–70, 84
Achari (Bihar program director), 171, 180
Ademola, Yemi, 27
Afghanistan, 83
Africa: Eradication Escalation effort in, 72–75, 85; mortality rates in, 7; smallpox transmission in, 38–39; surveillance and containment strategy in, 11; WHO eradication program in, 46–53. *See also* Nigeria
Akbar (Indian ruler), 88
American Management Association, 192
Anderson, James, 93
Andhra Pradesh (Indian state), 124
Anezanwu, A., 60–61, 67
Arora, R. R., 127
Assam (Indian state), 175, 176
assessment. *See* program evaluation
Atharva Veda (Hindo scripture), 89
attack phase, 98
Atutu Ochelebe, Lawrence, 35, 44, 183

Bangladesh, 11, 185
Banu, Rahima, 185

Basu, R. N., 97, 127, 153
belief in global eradication, 11, 26–27; program in Africa and, 47, 52–53; program in India and, 83–86, 161, 167–168. *See also* eradication of smallpox; surveillance and containment approach
Belkind, Myron L., 167
Bhattacharya, S., 143
bifurcated needle, 101–102, 109, 197, 205n30
Bihar (Indian state), 93, 177; decision by Minister of Health in, 169–172; new outbreaks compared (1974 and 1975), 176–177; political matters in, 157–161; surveillance and containment approach in, 106, 111–112, 115, 119, 140, 147–148; turning point in, 161–162, 163–164, 172, 173
biological warfare: defense against, 18, 195–196; suspicions of workers and, 159
Birmingham, England cases (1978), 186
Blair, Vachel, 24
Bohannan, Laura, 38–39
Brazil, 83, 84
Brilliant, Girija, 206n1
Brilliant, Larry, 129, 168, 206n1
Bulle, Wolfgang, 29, 30, 71

Calcutta, India, 93
Carro, Jean de, 92
cases, number of, as metric, 118–119
CDC. *See* Communicable Disease Center (CDC)
Central Africa, 72–75
Chandragupta (ruler in India), 88
chickenpox, 42, 154, 181
children: push for mass vaccination of, 171, 180; repeat vaccinations and, 93, 99; as search informants, 117, 148–149; vaccine in India and, 92–93
church missions: evacuation from Enugu and, 66–69; medical work by, 28; Ogoja outbreak and, 54–55, 57–58
Clara Swain Hospital in Uttar Pradesh, 139
Clark, William, 10
Cleveland, Harlan, 117
coalitions, 130–131, 189–190, 191
coercion, 206n1
Communicable Disease Center (CDC): author's position at, 84, 183; Bangladesh program and, 185; Epidemic Intelligence Service (EIS) training at, 18; eradication program in Africa and, 36–37, 46–53, 69, 72–73, 76, 77; managers in India, 131–134, 136, 160; name changes of, 200n2; oral history archive and, 206n5; smallpox eradication handbook of, 76; surveillance and containment approach at, 75–79; threat in New Mexico and, 19–22; WHO global program and, 84. *See also* Henderson, D. A.; Millar, Don; Sencer, David J.
communication, 130, 144, 191
community leaders, 45–46
Conrad, Lyle, 204n29
contagiousness of smallpox, 38
containment teams, 108–110, 115—117, 121
cowpox virus, 8–10, 92, 94
Cresswell, John, 93
cultural awareness: city life in Nigeria and, 43–45; foreign workers in India and, 110–111, 135–136, 138; importance of, 192; storytelling in Nigeria and, 62–63; village life in Nigeria and, 30–34, 43, 45–46; village wisdom about smallpox and, 74–75

detection of smallpox, 3–4, 77–78
Devi (Indian goddess), 89
Diesh, P., 125–126, 128, 130, 135–136, 145, 176–177
Directorate General of Helth Services (India), 103
district headquarters, 153–154
Dupont, 168

Durant, Will, 191
Dusthall, Anna, 92, 94
Dutta, Mahendra, 126, 130, 145, 169–172, 177, 180

Eastern Nigeria Ministry of Health, 59
EIS. *See* Epidemic Intelligence Service (EIS)
Emory University, 206n5
Enahoro, Peter, 67
Enugu, Nigeria: Eastern Nigeria eradication effort and, 43–44; wartime revisit to, 71
Epidemic Intelligence Service (EIS), 18
epidemiology, field of, 17–18
Eradication Escalation effort, 72–75, 85
eradication of smallpox: dream of, 8–11; origins of global program for, 10; proposed possibility for, 25–27; shift in primary strategy for, 53–59. *See also* belief in global eradication
Ethiopia, 185–186
Etzel, Ed, 160
evaluation teams, 154–155. *See also* program evaluation

Faith Tabernacle Church, 59
fetisheurs, 41–42
"field paranoia" syndrome, 167–168
financial support: cost in India and, 102; USAID and, 46; WHA and, 10, 47–48. *See also* government support; pharmaceutical philanthropy
firefighting analogy, 15–16, 58, 78, 118, 171–172
Foege, David, 64, 66, 67, 75
Foege, Michael, 37, 43, 88, 157–158
Foege, Paula, 64, 75, 78
Foege, Robert, 88
Foege, William (Bill): arrests and, 66, 70–71; car incidents and, 113, 114; early experiences with smallpox, 19–24; education of, 16–18; influences in youth of, 12–16; public health work in Africa and, 28–37; research in Tonga and, 24–25; shingles incident and, 114–115; study with Weller and, 25–27; T-shirt incident, 87. *See also* Foege family
Foege family: in Denver, 19; in India, 87–88, 137–138, 157–158, 183–184; in rural Nigeria, 29, 30–35, 37; in urban Nigeria, 43–44; wartime Nigeria and, 66–68, 71
foreign workers, 110–111, 135–136, 159
forms, 109, 110, 155–157, 197
Foster, Stan, 37, 73
Francis, Don, 139
fraud, 126–127

"Friday Afternoon Reflections" (newsletter), 47
Frost, Wade Hampton, 17–18

Gandhi, Indira, 111–112, 161
Gardner, Pierce, 24
Gates Foundation, 168, 205n30
Gelfand, Henry, 36–37, 69, 75, 84–85, 167, 205n2
GlaxoSmithKline, 168, 205n30
global health field, 17
Glokpur, George, 53
goddess of smallpox, 89–90, 96, 152
Government of India, 98–100, 110, 140; alliance with WHO, 129–131; support from, 102–103, 161, 167
government support: as critical, 190; in India, 102–103, 161, 167
Grasset, Nicole, 86, 87, 105, 106, 127–128, 129, 184
Gray, Herman, 35
Greenough, Paul, 206n1
Greenwald, Peter, 24

Harvard University, Department of Tropical Public Health, 26–27
Hawking, Stephen, 188
health education, 63
health workers, 73, 86, 102–103, 115; evaluation of personnel and, 137–139; "field paranoia" syndrome and, 167–168; strike by, 165–166; suspicions of, 159–161; tactical flexibility and, 190–191; training of, 59, 106–111. See also containment teams; search teams; special epidemiologists
Henderson, D. A., 19; CDC and, 24, 46, 202n5; program in India and, 86, 102, 164; surveillance and containment strategy and, 75; WHO eradication program and, 27, 30, 46, 48–49
Henderson, Ralph (Rafe), 204n29
herd immunity, 53, 74, 189. See also mass vaccination
history of smallpox, 5–8; in Africa, 39–42; in India, 88–92
Holwell, J. Z., 89, 91
Hopkins, Donald, 5–6, 73, 93, 94
households, 110, 151–153
human impacts of smallpox, 5–6
humility, value of, 192
Hunter, John, 8
Hunter, R. W., 93

index case, 17–18, 154
India, 11; beginnings of program in, 86–88; CDC managers in, 131–134; containment improvements in, 151–153; core alliance in, 129–131, 166; dissension in, 143–144; early vaccination efforts in, 92–97; first search in, 111–117; history of smallpox in, 88–92; key team members in, 123–127; last case in, 184; later searches in, 117–119, 147–148; main themes of program in, 122; monthly meetings and, 140–144, 169–172; nationwide programs in, 98–104; Operation Smallpox Zero in, 182–184; outbreaks compared (1974 and 1975), 176–177, 182, 184; rural vs. urban disparities in, 93, 96–97; scientific contributions of, 88–89; SEARO team in, 127–129; skepticism about strategy in, 83–86; smallpox goddess in, 89–90, 96; smallpox incidence in, 97, 100; special epidemiologists in, 134–140; strike by health workers in, 165–166; surveillance improvements in, 148–150; turning point in, 161–162, 163–164, 177. See also Bihar; Uttar Pradesh
Indian Council of Medical Research, 98
Indonesia, 83
injections, attitudes toward, 45. See also vaccination, resistence to
inoculation. See variolation
instruction sheets, 109, 156–157, 197
international community, assistance from, 11, 52. See also financial support; World Health Organization (WHO)
Ismach, Aaron, 50

James, S. P., 95
Jefferson, Thomas, 10
Jehan (Indian Shah), 88
Jenner, Edward, 8–10, 47, 92, 93
jet injector, 26, 45, 49, 50–52; vaccine dilution and, 24–25, 204n29
Jezek, Zdeno, 128
Johns Hopkins School of Hygiene and Public Health, 17–18
Joseph, N. (cook), 87, 137
Journal of International Health, 75

Kingma, Stuart, 133
Kohlstedt, Jim, 14
Kohlstedt, Shirley, 14

Lagos, Nigeria, 63–65, 64, 70, 71
Laney, Jim, 58
Langmuir, Alex, 18, 27
leadership effectiveness, 191
Lewis, Meriwether, 10
Lichfield, Mary, 44
Lichfield, Paul, 44, 58, 60, 70

Lincoln, Abraham, 7
Lucas, Adetokunbo, 63
Lutheran Church—Missouri Synod, 29
Lythcott, George, 201–202n1

Madhya Pradesh (Indian state), 106, 121, 176
maintenance phase, 98
Malin, Ali Maow, 186
management system in India, 133–134
mass vaccination: Abakaliki pilot project and, 58, 59; campaign in India and, 99–104; with other diseases, 78–79, 189; phases of, in India, 98; as primary strategy, 53–54, 59, 65–66, 74, 75–77; threat of return to, 169–172, 177, 180
Mather, Cotton, 41
Maulana Azad Medical College in Delhi, 124
McPherson, Dr., 94
measles, 38, 46–47, 72–73
Meiklejohn, Gordon, 114–115
Merck, 168, 205n30
metrics: belief in eradication strategy and, 161–162, 172; data analysis and, 145–147; evaluation criteria and, 154–155; number of outbreaks and, 118–119, 146, 161–162, 172, 182; number of vaccinations and, 93, 97; tracking of data and, 145–148. See also program evaluation
Millar, Don, 19, 37, 85, 132, 167; African eradication program and, 47, 69, 71, 72
Ministry of Health (India), 86, 123, 125, 166–167, 177, 180
Ministry of Health (Nigeria), 61, 66, 67–69
Montague, Lady, 41
morale, 99, 121, 138, 141, 142–143, 164, 172
Morris, Leo, 84
mortality rate, 6, 7, 10; in India, 91–92, 96, 97, 146
Moynihan, Daniel Patrick, 160–161
multiple pressure vaccination technique, 49

Narayan, J. P., 158
National Institute of Communicable Diseases (NICD), 86–87, 99–100, 102, 124, 204n27
Native Americans, 6, 7, 10
Nelmes, Sara, 8
New England Journal of Medicine, 25
New Mexico, smallpox threat in, 19–22
NICD. See National Institute of Communicable Diseases (NICD)
Nigeria, 28–42; eradication in Eastern region of, 60–72; fetisheurs in, 41–42; last case of

smallpox in, 73; possibility of eradication and, 27; smallpox in rural areas of, 37–39; surveillance and containment strategy in, 11, 60–72; variolation in, 40–42; village life in, 30–36; war in, 61–69; WHO eradication program in, 46–53
Nordstrom, Frank, 19
Norton, Charles, 93

Ogoja, Nigeria, outbreak, 54–59, 77, 79
Onitsha Bridge incident, 64–65
Operation Smallpox Zero, 182–184
optimism: unwarranted, 117; value of, 191. See also morale
oral histories, 206n5
Orissa (Indian state), 176
Ottemüller, Hector, 54
outbreaks: number of, as metric, 118–119, 146–147, 161–162, 172, 182; search results in Uttar Pradesh and, 113–114, 115, 173; transmission in Africa and, 38–39; variolation and, 40

Parasher, Umesh, 126
pathogen combinations, 36
Patna, Bihar, 158
Patwadangar. See Uttar Pradesh
Peace Corps, 27, 86
Ped-O-Jet, 50–51, 102
personnel. See health workers
Pfizer, 168
pharmaceutical philanthropy, 168, 205n30
PHC. See Primary Health Center (PHC)
Phipps, James, 8–9
physical effects of disease, 4–5
physicians, managerial skills of, 207n2
polio vaccine, 200n8
politics: Bihar's Minister of Health and, 169–172; climate in India and, 157–161; foreign workers and, 137, 159; risks to eradication program and, 61–69
Polybius (Greek historian), 52
population density, 8, 91, 99, 107
population size, 107
Precision Fabrics, 168
prevention: medical missions and, 28–29
Primary Health Center (PHC), 103, 108, 112, 119, 153–154
program evaluation, 99, 100, 192; assessments in India and, 100–102, 173–175; number of vaccinations, as measure, 93, 99; value of, 153–155. See also metrics
public health field, 17, 186–187; lessons from smallpox program for, 188–192
publicity, 166–167

quality control: evaluation system and, 154–155; monthly meetings in India and, 140–144; standards for vaccine and, 48–49, 104; training and, 108

Ramses V, 6, 89
Rao, A. R., 85, 134–135
Rao, C. K., 127
Ravenholt, Rei, 17, 18, 27, 200n1
Raya, Krishna, 88
recognition cards, 108, 109, 158
recordkeeping: containment in India and, 151, 155–157; early vaccination activities in India and, 93, 95, 96; forms and, 155–157; program in Uttar Pradesh and, 112
Reid, Gordon, 204n29
repeat vaccination, 93, 99, 100
reporting system: Africa and, 39; data tracking from, 145–147; forms and, 156; in India, 100, 103–104, 111, 112, 114, 117, 119
resource allocation, 191
reward system, 131, 181–182, 185
Richmond, Julius, 73
Ristad, Paula (wife of author), 16–17. See also Foege, Paula; Foege family
roadblocks, 61–63, 64–65
Roberto, Ron, 24
rotary lancet, 49, 50, 101
Rubin, Benjamin, 101

Sacco, Luigi, 92
Schweitzer, Albert, 15
Scott, Helenus, 92
search teams, 107–108, 148–150
SEARO. See Southeast Asia Regional Office (SEARO)
Sencer, David J., 84, 86, 132–133, 160, 183
Seva Foundation, 206n1
Shah Jehan. See Jehan (Indian Shah)
Sharma, M. I. D., 124–125, 126, 130, 145, 169–172, 176
shortcuts, 120
Shrivastav, J. B., 167, 177, 180
Shriver, Sargent, 27
SIDA. See Swedish International Development Authority (SIDA)
Sierra Leone, 73
Singh, Jit, 87, 88
Singh, Karan, 124, 135–136, 166, 177, 180
Singh, Mahendra, 127
Singh, Rajendra, 139–140
six-foot perimeter concept, 152–153
"Smallpox Zero," 87. See also Operation Smallpox Zero
Solex motorbikes, 54–55

Somalia, 186
South America, 7
South Asia, 83–84
Southeast Asia, 7–8
Southeast Asia Regional Office (SEARO), 86, 103, 105, 117, 135, 136; team members at, 127–129
South India, 85–86
special epidemiologists, 103, 117, 134–140, 142–143, 159–161
Steiger, Tony, 15
storytelling, 62–63
Strunk, Bill, 16
Stuart, Johannes, 133
supervision, 108
supplies, 63–65. See also vaccine
surveillance and containment approach: containment planning and, 108–110; in Eastern Nigeria, 60–72; efficiency of containment and, 162, 163, 174, 181; efficiency of searches and, 107, 120–121, 145, 154, 162, 166, 174; Eradication Escalation effort and, 72–75; history of, at CDC, 75–79; in India, 102, 105–122, 184 (see also India); indicators of containment and, 146, 161; nature of searches and, 107; personnel involved in, 106–111; reasons for effectiveness of, 77–79; search planning and, 107–108; as secondary strategy, 54, 75–77, 85; shift to, as primary strategy, 11, 73, 84–86; skepticism about, 83–86, 177, 180; smallpox bioterrorism and, 195–196; testing of, as primary strategy, 11, 60–72
Swain, Clara, 139
Swedish International Development Authority (SIDA), 131, 181–182

tactical flexibility, 190–191
take rates, 26, 100
talking drum, 45–46
Tamil Nadu, South India, 85
Tata Industries, 124, 168
tenacity, 191
terrorist threat, 195–196
Thompson, David, 44, 54–55, 58, 60, 70
Thompson, Joan, 44
Tonga research, 24–25, 26
training programs: EIS and, 18; for in India, 59, 106–111; special epidemiologists and, 136–137
Tranneus, J. E., 131
transmission of smallpox: decline in rate of, 162; endemic countries and, 72; epidemiological understanding and, 74–75; households and, 110; outbreaks in Africa and,

transmission of smallpox (continued)
38–39; risks of spread and, 56–57; sex trade
and, 205n2
travel: drivers and, 136–137; political matters
and, 157–161, 176–177; searches in India
and, 112–113, 114; spread of virus in Nigeria and, 67–68; WHO staff and, 129–130
trust, importance of, 190

underreporting, 39. See also reporting
system
UNICEF. See United Nations Children's
Fund (UNICEF)
United Lutheran Church of America, 28–29
United Nations, 52
United Nations Children's Fund (UNICEF),
104
United States: bioterrorism threat in, 195–
196; consultants from, 136 (see also foreign
workers; special epidemiologists); global
perspective and, 52, 132; smallpox in history of, 6–7; surveillance and containment
approach in, 195–196, 205n1
U.S. Agency for International Development
(USAID), 46, 47, 69, 72, 200n1
USSR, 48, 99, 104
Uttar Pradesh (Indian state), 139, 140; mortality rate in, 91–92; rise in numbers in,
147–148; surveillance and containment
approach in, 106, 111, 112–119; turning
point in, 162, 173–175; vaccine depot in,
95, 104

vaccination: benefits of, 93; as compulsory,
96; discovery of, 8–10; early efforts in
India, 92–97; resistence to, 59, 89, 91, 93–
94, 140, 153, 206n1; vs. variation, 40
vaccinations, number of, as metric, 93, 97
vaccination strategy: critical shift in, 11; in
nineteenth-century India, 93–96. See also
mass vaccination; surveillance and containment approach
vaccination teams: in Nigeria, 59; Peace

Corps volunteers and, 27. See also containment teams; health workers
vaccination techniques: advances in, 48–52,
101–102; dilution and, 24–25, 51; instruction sheet on, 109, 197; multiple pressure
vaccination technique, 49; in nineteenth-
century India, 94; possibilities for global
eradication and, 10. See also jet injector
vaccinators. See health workers
vaccine: delivery of, in India, 92–93; dilution
of, 24–25, 51; freeze-drying and, 104; production in affected countries, 10, 48, 94,
95, 104; sources of, 94, 99; standards for,
48–49, 104. See also supplies
vaccinia virus, 75
van Bibber, Dr. (Lincoln's physician), 7
variola minor, 185–186
variolation: development of, 40; in India, 89,
91, 95–96; Jenner and, 8–9; in Old World,
40–42

Washington, George, 6–7
watch guards, 152, 153
Watson, William, 133
Weller, Tom, 25–26, 200n8
West Africa, 72–75
West and Central African Smallpox Eradication/
Measles Control Program (CDC handbook),
76
West Bengal, India, 106, 121, 177
World Health Assembly (WHA), 10, 27, 47–
48, 98
World Health Organization (WHO), 10;
archival records and, 143–144; CDC
involvement and, 84, 160; Ethiopian
program and, 185–186; improvement
of tools and, 189; program in India and,
100–102, 104, 105, 117, 129–131, 155, 164;
program in Nigeria and, 46–53; surveillance and containment approach and, 74,
75–76. See also Southeast Asia Regional
Office (SEARO)
Wyeth Pharmaceuticals, 101, 205n30

Text: 10/14 Palatino
Display: Univers Condensed Light, Bauer Bodoni
Compositor: BookMatters, Berkeley
Indexer: Marcia Carlson
Cartographer: Bill Nelson